Judith Peek

# A DICTIO

# SUSS

## FOLK MEI

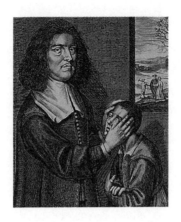

# A DICTIONARY OF
# SUSSEX
## FOLK MEDICINE

## Dr ANDREW ALLEN

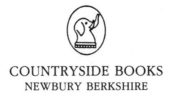

COUNTRYSIDE BOOKS
NEWBURY BERKSHIRE

Cover illustration: *Atropa Mandragora* from an
original illustration in the Mansell Collection

Title page illustration: *Valentine Greatrakes*. Line engraving, 1794.
(Wellcome Institute Library, London)

Designed by Mon Mohan
Produced through MRM Associates Ltd., Reading
Typeset by Paragon Typesetters, Queensferry, Clwyd
Printed by J.W. Arrowsmith Ltd., Bristol

# CONTENTS

# INTRODUCTION

The period of greatest interest to students of folk medicine in Sussex runs from the 16th to the mid-20th centuries. Before 1500 we have few sources specific to Sussex, and the boundaries, if any, between official and folk medicine are difficult to define. But it is clear that after 1500, particularly among poorer people the weakening of the Church's authority led to the growth of reliance on folk medicine.

The far-reaching authority of the medieval Church is undeniable. Its powerful mystique, means of consolation, and perpetual accompaniment through all the stages of life were allied to its organised charity and dense system of hospitals – at least 28 in Sussex – with specialised institutions such as leper hospitals. So far as we can tell, such influence provided a sort of universal spiritual and physical care system for both the souls and bodies of all its flock.

The secularization of large domains of society during the 15th-17th centuries, with the retreat of the Church into a more specialized role, created a division between a minority able to pay market prices for the services of licensed physicians and a majority who could not. Nor could they now turn to the Church for its healing magic (repudiated by Protestantism), consolation, and organized physical and spiritual support. This situation inevitably drove people to find alternative means of treatment and consolation in the form of self-help, folk medicine or alternative unlicensed practitioners.

By the mid-20th century, notably with the establishment of the National Health Service, the factors which had favoured the emergence and success of folk or popular medicine in the post-medieval period – namely the prohibitive cost of medical treatment and the incompetence of licensed doctors – had largely disappeared. The slow withering away of folk medicine in both rural and urban areas had, however, already begun in the 19th century with the spread of the rational scientific outlook. This succeeded in casting discredit not only on folk remedies which we can regard with the benefit of hindsight as bizarre, inefficacious and superstitious nonsense (for a

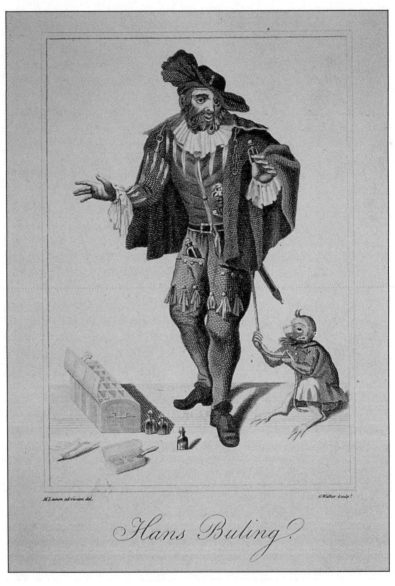

*Hans Buling from an engraving by G. Walker. This shows a typical mountebank holding a medicine bottle in his left hand and accompanied by a monkey. (Wellcome Institute Library, London)*

6

selection of the most bizarre see **Ague; Badger; Charms; Cow, Horse and Sheep; Curses, Spells and Witches; Fits; Gibbet; King's Evil; Lucky Stones; Mice; Runs of the Lights; Shrew Ash; Swallow Water; Thrush; Trees; Vipers/Viper-Catchers; Warts; Whooping Cough**) but also on many rural remedies which were of great and real efficacy (for example **Cobweb; Cunning Folk; Dog; Easter Bun; Egg; Elecampane; Flea/Fleabane/ Fleawort; Frog; Insects; Mould; Scurvy, Scurvy Grass, Samphire; Snails; Wormwood / Wormwort; Woundworts**).

Between the Church's retreat from its all-embracing role to the coming of the NHS most people in Sussex relied on folk medicine to cure their ills. Firstly, because professional medical treatment was of limited availability – most people in rural Sussex lived many miles from the nearest licensed doctor, in country where the tracks could be all but impassable with mud or snow for many months of the year.

Secondly, because licensed doctors were prohibitively expensive and had a well-justified reputation for bleeding their patients penniless. In the 17th and 18th centuries fees charged by doctors were usually of the order of £1-£30 per visit or short course of treatment; at the same period the average annual income of labourers, schoolmasters and carpenters was £4-£20 pa – figures which show that no more than the wealthiest 5-10% of the population, earning, say £70 pa or above could afford doctors (see **Earnings and the Affordability of Medicine**).

Thirdly, because the fortunate few who could afford to call in physicians weren't really so very fortunate. They were subjected to violent blood letting and purging, crude surgical techniques (operations carried out without anaesthetic or antiseptic precautions) and lethal chemical treatments based on concentrated sulphuric acid (the standard treatment for scurvy until the late 18th century) and salts of arsenic, lead, bismuth, antimony and mercury (the standard treatment for syphilis until the late 19th century). With such treatments, 16th to mid-19th century doctors probably killed more patients than they cured; one of the better documented cases being the frightful death of Charles II at the hands of his physicians.

The worst of the documented cases concerned fashionable, expensive doctors in or from London and large towns or resorts who treated the higher nobility or very wealthy patients with more money than sense. The small town doctors were rather more cautious and 'gentle', but the diaries and letters of well-to-do country people confirm that small town and village practitioners were generally regarded by contemporaries as dangerous, or incompetent, or both.

Many down-to-earth country folk who might have afforded the services of a doctor – yeomen, the better-off clergy, minor gentry, furriers, traders etc – weighed up the risks and benefits and placed their trust in homespun traditional remedies which, even if they weren't guaranteed to cure and didn't necessarily embody an immemorial wisdom, were seldom life-threatening. Indeed, much of our knowledge of folk medicine in 16th-18th century Sussex comes from the diaries, 'Receipt Books', household account books, and letters of literate educated people who sought out, for their own use, the best of the classical or traditional remedies described in herbals or used by their poorer non- or semi-literate neighbours.

Many of these remedies were handed down and exchanged within the rural community as part of their common heritage. When someone fell ill he might seek first of all to cure himself using either remedies traditional to his family, or recommended by friends or neighbours. If home treatment failed, or if the ailment fell into certain specific categories, he might turn to a 'white witch', 'wise woman', 'cunning woman' or 'cunning man', often skilled in herbal medicine, who might cure the ailment by prescribing a folk remedy, by therapeutic white magic, charms or spells (or the lifting of curses and spells inflicted by witches). More often it was a mélange of both.

Such individuals, based in the local community, commonly claimed to have a 'gift' for healing, either acquired or inherited. They operated in the context of a local economy and seldom asked for money for their services, preferring to be paid, tangibly or intangibly, in kind. 'Cunning folk' of both sexes were reputedly once as common as the parish clergy, and to be found in every parish in the country: 'Out of question they be innumerable which receive help by going to the cunning man or woman', lamented one pastor turned pamphleteer. The earliest mentions of cunning folk in Sussex are in the writings of Leonard Mascal of Plumpton Place and Andrew Borde of Pevensey during the reign of Henry VIII, and there were still 'wise women' in some Sussex villages as late as the 1920s-30s.

As many of their remedies were based on country herbs and practical psychology, it is probable that cunning folk brought about more cures than doctors who based their science on, say, the theory of the humours and who would often bleed or purge a patient as soon as look at him.

With the advances of medical science in the 19th century slowly raising public confidence in doctors and suspicion towards traditional rural charms and remedies, and with more zealous, systematic prosecution of unlicensed practitioners, cunning folk gradually retreated from their central place in the community into marginal quackery (small town cunning folk exploiting the gullible and superstitious for money) or the herbal treatment of minor ailments (see under **Cunning Folk – Grandmother Huggett's Cures**).

Most 16th to mid-19th century wise folk were respected members of the local community. But the too-cunning woman who sought money for her services, and who was prepared to exploit her knowledge of poisons and spells for evil as well as for, or instead of, benevolent ends, reputedly casting spells or poisoning cattle, was likely to be regarded as a witch, full stop. This reputation might cost her dear during periods of witch hysteria such as the 1560s-1680s when many cunning women with an ambiguous reputation, or lonely outcast old women who might come to be blamed for the ills of their neighbours, were lynched, ducked, or tried as witches (see **Curses, Spells and Witches**).

In towns such as Chichester, Midhurst, Petworth, Horsham, Arundel, Hailsham, Uckfield, Lewes, Battle, Hastings, Seaford and Rye, and in larger, more prosperous villages such as Cuckfield and Ditchling, apothecaries – forerunners of modern pharmacists – came to occupy an ambiguous position on the borderline between the official medicine of physicians and surgeons and the popular medicine of cunning folk, quacks, and self-help.

At the beginning of our period, in the 16th and 17th centuries, there were three rival bodies of licenced practitioners: 'physitians', who dated from the establishment of the Royal College of Physicians by Henry VIII, but never very common in the country in early times; surgeons/barber surgeons, who went through a confusion of incorporations until finally brought into order in 1797 by the establishment of the Royal College of Surgeons; and apothecaries, who after similar confusions had their status and prerogatives finally clarified by an Act of Parliament in 1815.

All three belonged to, and (in theory) were defended and regulated by trade bodies; and recognized in English law as being entitled to practise medicine – such practice, except for the treatment of certain specified conditons (the so-called 'Quack's Charter') being illegal if one did not belong to one or other of the recognized corporations.

The surgeons (initially aureoled with a traditional authority going back through the Middle Ages to the revered Ancients Galen and Hippocrates) were essentially specialists in surgical operations but – in practice, and especially in small towns and the countryside – functioned as general practitioners who also prepared their own drugs and potions.

The apothecaries (whose original aura of power and mystery had been imparted by their links with alchemy, poisons and mind altering substances) were specialists in the preparation and retailing of drugs, but in small towns and the countryside in practice they functioned as generalists who also carried out operations, which the surgeons as a corporation fought repeated court cases to prevent. The apothecaries brought similar actions to prevent surgeons from dabbling in general or internal medicine or preparing their own drugs, but the outcomes were invariably confused, and until well into the 18th century both surgeons and apothecaries were effectively family doctors and general practitioners.

As the 18th century progressed into the 19th however, there slowly emerged a patchy trend for surgeons and physicians to become the principal medical practitioners, and apothecaries as specialists in the preparation and retailing of drugs – a de facto state of affairs which passed into law with the Act of 1815.

It is not entirely clear whether this represented a 'victory' for the surgeons and physicians, or an inevitable division of labour between practising doctors who no longer had the time to seek out and prepare drugs (though some did continue to produce and even retail their own medicines until 1815 and beyond) and apothecaries/pharmacists who found trading in and preparing drugs so profitable and time-consuming that they no longer had the necessary skills to function effectively as medical practitioners, though they remained prescribing pharmacists and occasional medical practitioners and were not yet the 'pure' pharmacists of today.

So, from being generalists who possessed an *officina* for the preparation and sale of drugs, apothecaries became primarily manufacturers and retailers of drugs, increasingly occupying an ambiguous position on the borderline between licensed and unlicensed medicine: preparing drugs for surgeons and physicians and dispensing drugs prescribed by them. But they also imported, prepared and retailed an incredible range of drugs of ancient repute, exotic origin or modern discovery for use in self-medication, the preparation of folk medicines or even the poisoning of a spouse.

They revelled too in dispensing their often arcane, esoteric and forbidden knowledge, counselling and prescribing; occupying a zone of indeterminate dimensions between the licensed medicine of surgeons and physicians and the alternative world of self-help, wise women, mountebanks and quacks. They prepared in their vats, mortars and stills and dispensed from their jars and vials – bezoard, camphor, catholicon, castoreum, asphodel, garlic, sal ammoniac, white wine vinegar, anocardium, aquae vitae, aristolochia, Jesuit's bark, balsam, borage, betony, viper oil, viper fat, snake sloughs, tincture of opium, acacia, fly agaric, anise, scurvy grass pills, samphire, gum arabic, fresh and dried herbs of every description, rosy tinted soporifying pain-killing laudanum, ether, salts of antimony, lead, mercury, arsenic and absinthe.

They also provided exotica such as myrrh, theriac, amber, cardamon, cubebs, mummy, requies magna, Spanish fly, mandrakes and false mandrakes, jars of live leeches and, from the mid-18th century, the first brand-name medicines with a

11

local, regional or national distribution, advertised in broadsheets or in the newspapers which had recently come into existence.

Medicinal herbs, if not grown in the physic or cottage garden, could also be bought from 'herb women' who either collected herbs in the countryside for sale to fellow villagers, to the Big House, or to apothecaries; or acted as intermediaries for growers or apothecaries, crying their wares from door to door through villages and towns.

Charlatans, cancer doctors, mountebanks, saltimbanques, merry andrews and quacks passed through every hamlet, village and town at frequent intervals and – together with ballad singers, bear wards, buffoons, clowns, comedians, conjurors, geomancers, hocus pocus men, jugglers, mandrake men, minstrels, puppet masters, rope dancers, toad-eaters, tooth drawers and tumblers – formed part of the colourful scene at fairs and markets. Charlatans travelled the countryside on foot, on horseback or in a simple horse-drawn carriage, selling potions, pills or powders guaranteed to cure every disorder. Mountebanks (from the Italian *montem banco*, to mount on a bench or stage) and saltimbanques were grander charlatans who dressed in fine black velvet clothes and travelled in horse-drawn carriages. At each stopping place they set up a stage in front of their mobile consulting rooms and with a more elaborate selling spiel, put on a show with tumblers tumbling and toad-eaters swallowing toads.

Merry andrews were charlatans or mountebanks whose acts might include comedy, broad humour, and singing and dancing. Their prototype, reputedly, was 'Merry' Andrew Borde of Pevensey, lapsed Carthusian monk, physician to Henry VIII, versifier, traveller, author of serious and thoughtful medical works (*A Breviary of Health*, etc) and compilations of bawdy sub-Rabelaisian tales, accused by his many enemies within the medical establishment of being a *montem banco* (which he undoubtedly was) and of running a brothel in Southampton (which may have been a trumped-up charge).

Unlike the cunning man or woman or white witch, who often possessed genuine skills in traditional medicine and practical psychology, and who could not afford to trick, at least

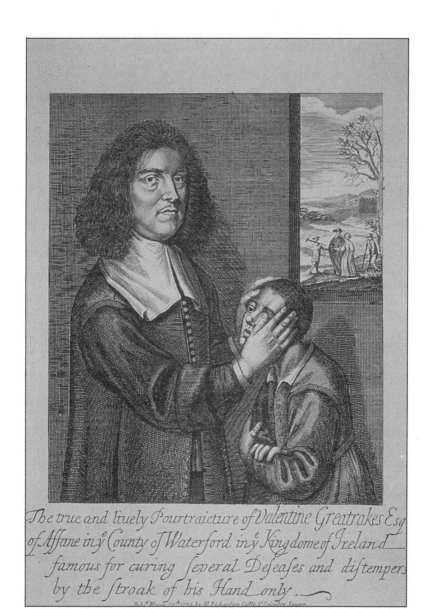

The true and truely Pourtraicture of Valentine Greatrakes Esq
of Affane in ye County of Waterford in ye Kingdome of Ireland
famous for curing several Deseases and distempers
by the stroak of his Hand only.

13

consciously and knowingly, the family and neighbours among whom he or she would have to pass their life, charlatans and mountebanks were undoubtedly in the business of duping the gullible of their money, but their marvellous elixirs and potions were less expensive than the treatments of conventional doctors and usually less dangerous. Less expensive, however, doesn't mean cheap. In his diary entry for the 9th July 1760, Thomas Turner of East Hoathly, Sussex, writes:

'In the afternoon my wife walked to Whitesmith to see a mountybank and his toad-eaters perform wonders, who has a stage built there, and comes once a week to cuzen a parcel of poor creatures of their money by selling his packets, which is to cure people of more distempers than they ever had in their lives, for 1s each'.

This at a time when the average rural wage was of the order of 2-3s a week. Then, as now, people were willing to suspend disbelief and to pay outrageous sums for remedies which promised rejuvenation, a cure for baldness or impotence or relief from chronic ill-health.

After travelling the roads the charlatan/mountebank often settled down – perhaps for a few weeks before setting off again, perhaps permanently – took rooms and opened a 'practice' in a well-situated market town such as Chichester, Horsham or Lewes. Towns provided a fertile ground for quackery because almost everyone was ill most of the time, the poor and not-so-poor could not afford the services of licensed doctors and, removed from their rural roots, were cut off from much of the lore and wisdom embodied in rural folk remedies, cut off from the advice of wise women and cunning men (in towns, the profession of a cunning man or woman existed but was shaded into that of the profit-oriented quack). Impotent suffering or recourse to a quack were the only two available options in the face of serious illness.

The heyday of the quack was in the period 1600-1800. For two centuries, mountebanks and quacks competed with, and often outcompeted, the lumbering, frequently pompous, licensed physicians, setting up consultancies and openly advertising their services. Thereafter, they were slowly forced into more marginal territory; as the skills of the official medics improved and became relatively better value so the noose of official regulations tightened around the quacks' throats, forcing them to function in grey areas or clandestinely.

In theory, laws dating from the reign of Henry VIII had restricted medical practice to licensed surgeons, physicians and apothecaries, allowing unlicensed people to treat only a very limited range of ailments. But in the early days at least there were relatively few cases of licensed practitioners, or the civil authorities, pursuing or prosecuting cunning folk or quacks; those recorded almost invariably involved fashionable high-profile quacks setting up in towns in direct competition to licensed practitioners, and poaching a wealthy clientele.

Justices – who may not have shared the licensed practitioners' inflated estimates of their own competence – were markedly reluctant to arouse popular indignation by encouraging the pursuit or conviction of cunning folk who were often well thought of in their communities, widely regarded as possessing healing skills at least equal to those of licensed practitioners, and who posed no evident threat to public health or order. The justices were also reluctant or unable to pursue travelling quacks who again were popular figures, and who inhabited a marginal world of here-today-gone-tomorrow domains largely beyond the reach of the still short and local arm of the English law.

In approaching the material in this book, it is important to avoid the two equally misguided, mutually symmetrical prejudices so many people have or develop when they hear the words 'folk' or 'rural' medicine.

The first is the notion that the corpus of folk or rural medicine embodies a largely lost immemorial handed-down medical wisdom in every way superior to modern scientific medicine because it was gentler, more traditional and more humane. The second prejudice or error is the opposite notion, held by most 19th and early to mid-20th century scientists and medics as well as by most other people, that folk

15

medicine was nothing but a farrago of ignorance and absurd superstition.

There is some truth behind both prejudices. I have already indicated that many of the old Sussex folk cures really did work, and 19th and 20th century medicine would have progressed much more rapidly if doctors and scientists had kept an open mind and been willing to learn from folk practice, rather than dismiss the whole en bloc as superstitious silliness. Whether such remedies were the discoveries of English country people, or whether they worked their way into the rural community via Anglo-Saxon, medieval and early modern translations of Greek and Roman authors isn't easy to discover – except for example, when a herb was introduced to Britain in say, the Middle Ages for medicinal purposes, where the origin of the knowledge is clearly exotic.

On the other hand, a summary dip through the entries that follow reveals as much or more that is 'superstitious nonsense', reflecting the practices of what was in some ways a backward society with a gullible, disorientated populace desperate to try out, and believe in, any remedy which promised relief from pain and suffering.

The balanced truth is that the one unifying feature of the period of folk medicine is its – utterly glorious – heterogeneity; compared with the much greater coherence of the medieval medicine which preceded it and modern medicine.

Medieval medicine was articulated around two stable poles: a small corpus of medical knowledge and theory based on the works of a limited number of classical authors such as Galen; and the medieval Catholic Church which, with its powerful magic, concerned itself with the physical as well as the moral health of the community – though it saw no difference between physical and moral health. The former they saw as a reflection of the latter – providing hope for the suffering and solace for the dying, and an ordered framework within which people could live, grow old and die within a shared community and, relatively speaking, without fear.

From the 15th century onwards the great edifice of the medieval world began to crumble and fall apart. The discovery and translation of new Greek and Roman medical texts and later the development of scientific medicine replaced the stable corpus and practices of medieval medicine with a continuously changing succession of new theories, practices and fashions. With the Reformation, the Church largely withdrew from the field of sickness and health and its claim to a powerful magic, leaving an enormous vacuum and its flock helpless and alone in the face of misery and disease.

Eventually, this vacuum would be largely filled by scientific medicine, together with modern complementary practices such as homeopathy, acupuncture, and so forth. But from the 16th until into the 19th or early 20th century official medicine could not fill the vacuum left by the withdrawal of the medieval Church. It was too expensive for most of the population; its sometimes dangerous and always changing theories and practices invited legitimate scepticism and fear – so most people in both the countryside and towns had to fend for themselves.

The more educated, particularly in the still small but slowly growing middle class, put together their own programmes of treatment by exploring as discriminatingly as possible both the knowledge in herbals and other medical texts and the traditional practices of the communities in which they lived.

The rural and urban poor made up 70-80 per cent of the population but, being less educated and mainly illiterate, they were not in a position to show the same selectivity. Certainly they made use, often to good effect, of whatever healing lore was traditional in their family or community, but in the desperation of illness and looming death were understandably ready to try out any – *any* – remedy which promised salvation. This could be the distorted memory of some old cure once current in the Middle Ages, or it might reflect age-old primitive patterns of thought about the causes of disease and the logic of treating illness or even the garbled thrice-distorted hearsay about a cure which had worked in the next village. They would also turn to anyone who was reputed to have or claimed to have healing skills, whether wise woman, cunning man, or mountebank. So we have the fascinating heterogeneity which is the one unifying feature of folk medicine in Sussex between the 16th and 20th centuries.

In the entries of this Dictionary I have tried to give a multitude of glimpses into, or vignettes of, life in Sussex during this period. In view of the patchiness of the source material, composed as it is mainly of glimpses, I have not intended or attempted any kind of deep analysis of the history and social context of folk medicine in Sussex. Such would require quite another book, drawing on contextual material from the rest of Britain and Europe. But where appropriate I have given a necessary minimum of context; explaining, where it is possible to explain, the origins of a particular remedy and the reasons why some remedies really did work. I have also indicated the patterns of thought or view of the working of the Universe which made it seem natural and logical to treat an illness in a way which from our modern viewpoint would seem illogical and bizarre.

Dr Andrew Allen
Findon Valley, Worthing
September, 1995

# AGUE

Ague – malaria: 'the quakes', 'Old Johnny Axey', 'Lord John's Fever' in Sussex dialect – used to be endemic in marshy areas of the county such as the Bosham, Selsey and Pagham Marshes in the west; Amberley Wild Brooks and the Arun Marshes from Littlehampton to Stopham; Adur Marshes; Lewes Levels and Ouse and Cuckmere Marshes; The Mountney, Pevensey, Manxey, Glynleigh, Horse Eye and Hooe Levels; and the Pett, Guldeford, Walland and Romney Marshes on the Kent/Sussex borders near Rye.

Everyone living in or near the marshes – which once covered more than a quarter of Sussex – suffered from malaria. In the 16th-18th centuries the average life expectancy at birth in villages in the Sussex, Kent and Essex marshes was 14 years, against 35 for the rest of England (for comparison: around 50-55 in late Victorian England, 70 + today). Those who moved into the marshes succumbed even more rapidly than the relatively resistant locals; a situation reflected in a traveller's tale repeated in several Sussex sources during the 18th century. It had apparently been lifted or 'adapted' from Daniel Defoe's account of his travels in the Essex marshes, but it seems that he in turn had lifted and adapted a tale circulating in many of the marshy areas of England, including Sussex. Passing through the Sussex marshes the traveller was informed by a local that:

'There was a farmer nearby, who was then living with his five and twentieth wife, and his son had already had a dozen. The reason, as the merry fellow told me, who said he had had about a dozen and half of wives himself (tho' I found afterwards he fibbed a bit) was this: that they being bred on the marshes themselves and season'd to the place did tolerably well with it; but that they always went up into the Wild (ie Weald) for a wife; that when they took their young lasses out of the wholesome and fresh air, they were healthy, fresh, and clear, but when they came out of their native air into the marshes among the fogs and agues and damps, that they presently changed their complexion, got an ague or two, and seldom held it above half a year, or a year at the most; and then said he, merrily, we go to the hills again and fetch another.'

But while mortality from malaria was highest in the marshes, most people in Sussex lived within a mosquito's flight of a stagnant pool or *Anopheles*-infested swamp. It is impossible to estimate the proportion of the population with malaria, but from the high incidence of deaths linked to 'agues', and from the remarks of 17th and 18th century Sussex diarists – all of whom either suffered from ague or mention family, neighbours or friends with ague – it seems that between a third and two thirds of the population suffered from malaria in either a mild or a severe form.

Here, for example, is the Revd Giles Moore, Rector of Horsted Keynes (a village high in the Weald between Lewes and East Grinstead, many miles from the lowland marshes), writing in his diary in March 1667:

'my ague, being an each day ague, came againe, and held me till the 19th. I payd Dr Parker for coming over from Rotherfield to see mee £1. I gave Goodwyfe Ward, for being necessary to mee, 1s, and I payd Mr Duke, curate of Pricomb for preaching one whole Sunday, hee also staying 5 dayes in my house 10s.'

And Walter Gale, schoolmaster of another Wealden village, Mayfield, on the 14th January 1750:

'In passing the Star (Inn) I met with Mr Eastwood, we went in and spent 2d apease. Fitness the Miller was there, from whom I learned that 20 drops of the spirits of hartshorn in half a quartern of gin will drive away ague: he allowed that he has driven his many a time.'

Spirit(s) of Hartshorn was either a potentially dangerous aqueous solution of ammonia, originally obtained by rasping/slicing/calcining and macerating or distilling harts' antlers; used as the base of many medicines and, because of its association with stags, believed to have powerful aphrodisiac and medicinal virtues. Or – and perhaps more likely in this context – a macerate or distillate of the buckhorn or hartshorn plantago *Plantage coronopus*, widely used against ague, often in the form of a cataplasm applied to the wrists. Sometimes the whole plant, roots included, was hung round the neck as an amulet.

And Mr Thomas Marchant of Little Park, Hurstpierpoint:

'May 10th 1727. At Lewes; and came home sick. It proved to be ague, of which I had several fits. It held to the 19th, on which day I first mist it . . . '
'March 26th 1728. Marrian set out for Oxford to bring J. Marchant home, on account of the small pox, which is much there. Mr Marten laid up here with an ague.'

And the Revd John Allin, Vicar of malarial Rye, merchant, speculator, and dabbler in alchemy and astrology, in a letter to his friend Mr Phillip Fryth, surgeon-apothecary. On 24 February 1664 he has

'gotten a greate ague wich shooke me last nyght an hour, but was pretty crancke [brisk] this morning'. [On 2 March] 'all the last weeke I was so ill I could not enjoy my selfe, much less doe buisines: I had 2 greate shaking fitts of an ague on thursday and saturday nyght last weeke; ye last nyght of wich I had 2 watch't with me, and I sweate lustily for 10 houres; since yt I have mist my ague through mercy, but cannot get my cold and cough away yet.'

And John Baker of Horsham, in a diary entry dated 25 February 1773:

'was taken with a violent ague – drank hot punch and Madeira negus – found myself heavy with that . . . Slept well most of night: drank much milk and water, wonderfully refreshing – which sat pleasantly on my stomach'.

From 26 February to 10 March Mr Baker suffered severe agues and was treated by the local doctor Mr Reid.

And finally an extract from Mary Capper's diary relating her stay at Wilmington, at the foot of the Downs, near the Cuckmere marshes, from November 1781 to October 1782:

'Marsh 21st. Sat a few minutes with a neighbour, Mrs King. She has been afflicted with an ague for several months and her children are in the same pitiable condition. Agues are frequent here, and very difficult to remove.'

Malaria began to give ground from about 1790 and by 1900 had disappeared from most of Sussex, except for the Pett, Guldeford and Romney Marshes on the Sussex/Kent borders where it lingered until as recently as the 1920s. This was not because of advances in medical knowledge, or any calculated plan to eradicate the *Anopheles* mosquitos which act as vectors for the malarial *Plasmodium*; the cause of malaria, vaguely associated with the *mal aria* or unwholesome air of swampy districts, was still unknown. It appears, simply, that drainage schemes during the late 18th and the 19th centuries converting marshes into water meadows or agricultural land had reduced the *Anopheles* to densities so low that mosquitos could no longer serve as an effective vector for the malarial parasite.

For our Sussex ancestors, malaria was effectively incurable. Of course, the relatively efficacious anti-malarial drug quinine had been discovered and was in sporadic use in Europe by the 17th century. But the only source of the Cinchona bark from which it was extracted was in the Spanish Empire in the New World and the trade in quinine was a monopoly controlled by the Jesuits, so many patriotic English people refused to import, sell or buy the despised – and for most pockets prohibitively expensive – 'Spanish' or 'Jesuit's Bark'. Through the 17th and 18th, and in rural areas into the 19th, centuries, Sussex people 'drew' or 'drove' their agues as best they could with age-old remedies – the most widespread and bizarre of which involved swallowing live spiders.

In fever-ridden areas of Sussex, sufferers used to swallow these rolled in butter to draw their agues. Sometimes the spider was taken with bread or breadcrumbs. In 1745, for example, Dr Richard Meade wrote from Rye to a friend in London with advice on curing agues. Among the cures he suggested was this, common in the marshland villages around Rye:

'take a Spyder alive, cover it with new soft crummy Bread without bruising it; let the Patient swallow it fasting.'

Another remedy was 'a spyder gently bruised and wrapped up in a raisin or spread upon bread and butter.'

In his book on British spiders, Bristowe (1958) describes an afternoon spent with a lady during which they both sampled various species of spider to see which of them tasted the best. For readers who may wish to indulge in this gastronomic delight and imagine themselves back into the world of their 18th century forbears, he records that the orb web spider *Aranaeus quadratus*, the largest British spider, came out on top with its 'slightly nutty flavour'. It can't be worse than eating snails or oysters can it?

Another spider recipe is given by John Goodyer, the Petersfield botanist, writing in 1624:

'The spyder being wrought into One masse with a plaister, and spread upon linen and soe layed to ye forehead and temples doth cure the periodicall circuits of tertian agues.'

Other cures involved wearing spiders. In the 17th and 18th centuries sufferers used to wear a plump live spider imprisoned in a nutshell or muslin bag suspended around the neck.

Using spiders to cure agues was not so illogical as it might seem to our modern way of thinking. Much early medicine was based on two overlapping principles. First, the 'homeopathic' principle that like is drawn to like, hence that the shivery, shiver-inducing spider could be used to draw out or act as a suitably attractive scapegoat for the transference of the shivering ague, so vividly described in the Sussex saying 'Old Johnny Axey's running his finger down my back', with its parallel in the shivers one feels when a spider runs over one's flesh. Second, the Doctrine of Signatures, whereby the form, markings or behaviour of animals and plants were signatures, clues or signs from God, or whatever powers had made the world, indicating their medicinal use. Hence, the shivery, vibratory nature of spiders was self-evidently a signature indicating that they might be useful as a cure for shivery agues. In the same way the heart-shaped leaves of the woodsorrel were a sign that it had been placed here below as a cure for heart disease and the pulmonary markings of the lungwort a sign that its role in the scheme of things was as a cure for pulmonary disease.

The shivering and trembling of the aspen – Latin name *Populus tremula*; Sussex names Old Wives' Tongues, Quackin' Ash, Shakin' Asp – was, equally clearly, a signature. Throughout Sussex, people drank infusions of aspen against ague (a cure which could only have had magical virtues, as the aspen is devoid of any chemical principles effective against malaria) or used a variety of procedures to transfer their agues to an aspen tree. We know that it was the special shivering quality of the aspen that was important here, because there are no records at all of people transferring their agues to hazels, oaks, birches, etc. For example, one Sussex writer's nurse during her childhood towards the end of the 19th century 'had seen a man unwinding lengths of rope which he had coiled round his body on to an aspen, as he ran round and round its trunk, singing:

"Ague, ague, I thee defy;
Ague, ague, to this tree I thee tie" '

This is a clear case of transference magic; the disease was being ritually 'given' to the aspen. The nurse who had seen this done firmly believed that one could indeed rid oneself of ague by this method 'if you knew the way'. Another writer records a different method of transferring ague to an aspen. You must take clippings from the sufferer's finger and toe nails while he is asleep, without his knowing (a restrictive condition!), and also cut hair from the nape of his neck; you must wrap them in paper and put them in a hole in an aspen tree.

A popular charm against ague widely used in the 18th and 19th centuries, recorded among others by the Revd W.D. Parish, ran as follows:

'Ague, ague, I thee defy! Three days shiver, Three days shake; Make me well for Jesus's sake!'

There is an element of realistic prognosis here. Malaria is normally an intermittent disease which may well clear up of its own accord after a few days – three in the case of the most common 'tertian' form – but the patient also assisted nature by the magical procedure of writing the charm on a three-cornered piece of paper and wearing it round his neck until it dropped off. Three, always a powerful number, here more particularly symbolizes the three days of shivering and shaking; and may also have invoked the Trinity, often symbolized by a triangle.

But while spiders, aspens and charms are frauds with no real efficacy against malaria, the people of the herbal era were not wholly defenceless against their agues. Country people in marshy districts of Sussex drank infusions of willow bark to treat the complaint. Willow bark contains precursors of, and was the original source of, acetyl salicylic acid, the active ingredient of aspirin. Willow bark 'aspirin' wasn't a cure for malaria, but would have helped alleviate some of its symptoms.

A second plant used against ague fevers was feverfew: the fever foe or fever fugue, for putting fevers to flight, whether the fever was malaria (cf the Cornish *les derth*, ague plant) plague, or simply 'flu. As a fever fugue it was grown in physic and cottage gardens across Sussex. Again, not a cure for malaria, but capable of alleviating malarial symptoms.

Finally, a cure which falls into the – very! – miscellaneous category. *The Gentleman's Magazine* in the 1730s reported that the trial had come on at Lewes 'of a Soldier who pretended to cure a Boy of the Ague; and thinking to frighten it away, by firing his Piece over the Boy's Head, levell'd it too low and shot his Brains out.'

See also **Cobweb** and **Trees.**

# BADGERS

Badger oil and fat massaged into the scalp were popular Sussex cures for thinning or receding hair or baldness. The principle here is plainly that of sympathetic magic: by rubbing in preparations made from the hirsute badger one might rub in and and assimilate the secret of its hairiness.

Badger fat was also used to treat coughs, shortness of breath, rheumatism, sprains and strains.


# BIRCH WINE, A Recipe For

Gerard (*An Herball or Generall Historie of Plantes*, 1597) says 'Concerning the medicaments and medicinale use of the Birch tree or his parts, there is nothing extant either in the old or new writers'.

However, in a curious work entitled *A collection of above Three hundred Receipts in Cookery etc. for the use of Good wives, Tender mothers and Careful Nurses — by several Hands. Printed for Mary Kettleby 1728*, one finds the following 'receipt' for a diuretic laxative tonic cordial Birch Wine, 'as made in Sussex':

'Tak sap of Birch fresh drawn, boil it as long as any scum arises; to every Gallon of Liquor put two pounds of good Sugar; boil it half an Hour and scum it very clean; when tis almost cold, set it with a little yeast spread on a Toast; let it stand five or six days in an open Vessel, stirring it often; then take such a Cask as the Liquor will be seen to fill; and fire a large Match dipt in Brimstone, and put it into the Cask, and stop in the Smoak, till the match is extinguish'd, always keeping it shook, then shake out the ashes, and, as quick as possible, pour in a pint of Sack or Rhenish, which taste you like best, for the Liquor retains it; rince the Cask well with this, and pour it out; Pour in your Wine, and stop it close for six Months, then, if 'tis perfectly fine, you may Bottle it.'

In the Highlands, notably in the Cairngorms around Aviemore, birch wine tonic was made by crofters and cottagers until at least the 1890s, but I have not heard of it being made in Sussex after the 18th century.

## BRACKET FUNGUS

This fungus, also known as amadou, held a favoured place among Sussex cottage remedies. Circular pads with holes in the middle (two are illustrated in the *Sussex County Magazine* No. 6, 1932, p709) were said to make the most comfortable of corn plasters; while in cases of bleeding a slice was used as a styptic.

For other treatments for bleeding, see **Cobweb, Cunning Folk: Grandmother Huggett's Cures, Dog, Egg, Elecampane, Frog, Moulds, Snails, Woundworts.**

## CHARLATANS, MOUNTEBANKS AND QUACKS
**Three Portraits:**

### 1. MESSRS BRUNSWICK AND TOURNEFORT

The popular doctors of the 17th and 18th centuries were the travelling quacks who were in competition with the regular practitioners. These quacks would visit a small country town for two or three months, travel on through the countryside visiting fairs and markets, and then stop in another town for a few months, especially during the winter when the impassable Sussex 'roads' made travelling virtually impossible, hampered even more by belongings and baggage.

Among the most popular of those travelling through Sussex in the last quarter of the 18th century – if we go by their own self publicity in local newspapers, and the frequency with which they are mentioned in other sources – were Messrs Brunswick and Tournefort. According to statements published in local newspapers, these two effected some remarkable cures. Among their miracles was the healing of John Mellish, a servant of one Ibbotsen of Arundel, who suffered from 'a dropsy in the stomach' and promptly celebrated his cure by advertising it in the local paper, probably at the instigation of Brunswick and Tournefort, who may have paid him. Furthermore, the son of George Lane, also of Arundel, was cured by them of the 'tertian ague' (see **Ague**) and 'fever and complement of worms' (see **Wormwood**), after applying in vain to regular practitioners for relief. Similarly, 'Ann Barnard, at the sign of the Coach and Horses in Marling, nr Chichester', had been subject to 'a decay of sight' for many years, and had the melancholy prospect of becoming blind when, fortunately, she came across Messrs Brunswick and Tournefort and became 'properly cured'. Henry Hawkins of the Parish of Climping had been afflicted with the 'Cholicky Disorder for a twelvemonth' when the duo got hold of him and set him to rights.

All these patients gave their testimony in the local paper, with their signature or mark attached. They were further supported by Thomas Pennycud (an old version of Pennicott, formerly a common Sussex name) who complained of 'pains in the stomach so severe that he could not keep his victuals down' until Brunswick and Tournefort relieved them.

But these cases pale into insignificance before that of John Ide, labourer, of Boxgrove, who testified that these two remarkable healers had cured him of leprosy, the testimony being signed by John Ide himself, and John Tubb and Henry Southward, overseers of that parish. Nor was this the only case of leprosy to be successfully treated. On 3rd December 1771 the public could read the following notice in the *Lewes Journal*:

'This is to acquaint the PUBLIC that I, ELIZABETH BURCHETT, of Shier, near Guildford, aged 50 years, have for the space of 15 years laboured under a violent leprosy, which covered my whole body with a most Foetid Scab; I was continually confined to my chair without finding the least repose by Day or Night; I had recourse to Doctors of superior Note, but no good accrued to me for the consultations; they unanimously declared that my Case was desperate, whichever I have found not to be so; for with the help of God, and the two Doctors Brunswick and Tournefort, I do declare, in this publick manner, that I was perfectly cured in a space of four months; I am now free from all Pain. My Body is entirely healed; and for a confirmation of the Truth of what I have asserted, I have given the Present under my Hand in the Presence of the undermentioned witnesses.'

The declaration is signed Elizabeth Burchett, John Burchett, her husband, and Thomas Gibbs.

\* \* \* \*

## 2. DR FLUGGER

All that seems to be known about Dr Flugger is that he was the inventor or 'Author of Lignorum Anti-Scorbutic Drops' (scorbutic pertaining to scurvy, with rickets one of the commonest deficiency diseases in pre-modern England); and the record of some remarkable cures attributed to that wonderful remedy. He seems to have been remembered with gratitude in Horsham, from where Mr Richard Cook, a cooper by trade, addressed the following letter to the *Sussex Advertiser and Lewes Journal* in December 1770:

'To Dr FLUGGER, Author of the Lignorum Anti-Scorbutic Drops.
   Sir,
   I should be guilty of ingratitude to you, and injustice to my fellow creatures, were I not to make public the surprising cure my wife hath received in taking 8 bottles of your Lignorum Anti-Scorbutic drops.
   After having been afflicted upwards of sixteen years with several ulcers in her legs, which, notwithstanding every method that could be thought of was tried, and no expense spared, became very foul and corrupted; insomuch that a mortification was hastily ensuing, and a violent Fever had seized her, together with a whole complication of disorders;

so that her life was really miserable, and all relief dispaired of but by death; till prescribed by Mr Sheubridge, the agent for the sale in this town, to try your Drops, which to the surprise of all who know her, and much to our comfort, perfected a Cure in a few months; and she is now in perfect health and free from all disorders whatever.

    Witness my hand,
        Richard Cook, Cooper.
        Horsham December 22, 1770.
PS – The truth of this may be relied upon, and can be testified by many of the inhabitants of this town...'

It would be interesting to know whether Dr Flugger's miraculous Lignorum Anti-Scorbutic Drops contained, as they may well have done, ingredients such as scurvy grass or samphire, which have genuine anti-scorbutic properties.

\*    \*    \*    \*

## 3. CHEVALIER TAYLOR, The

It must have been a great day for Lewes when, in August 1761, the Chevalier Taylor, celebrated itinerant oculist, arrived in town for the purpose of curing those with defective sight.

His visit was preceded by the distribution of an advertisement in verse form originally printed in Tunbridge on 21 August 1758. 'On a Child born blind, and who yesterday received his sight in the Presence of all the Nobility, by the Chevalier John Taylor', the copy of which exists in the Sussex Archaeological Society's valuable collection of 18th century Lewes advertisements and broadsides:

Taylor's visit to Lewes was also announced beforehand in the *Sussex Weekly Advertiser*. He stayed at the White Hart, then as now a famous Lewes hostelry. On 24 August 1761 the paper announced:

'Exactly at 11 o'clock this morning, as usual in all parts of the world, the poor afflicted in the eye may have his best assistance free and the faculty and gentry are invited to be

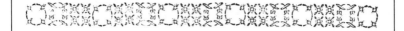

TUNBRIDGE, *Aug.* 21, 1758.

## On a Child born Blind, and who Yefterday receiv'd his Sight in the Prefence of all the Nobility, by the Chevalier T A Y L O R.

FROM Cure to Cure the Chevalier,
  Quick as his Tongue, does Wonders here :
Beneath his Hand, with hideous Cries,
Through Fear not Pain, an Infant lies ;
But in few Minutes blefs'd with Sight,
Now ftarts aftonifh'd at the Light ;
The Light that, as with Magic Pow'r,
Prefents a World unknown before :
With painful Pleafure fighs awhile,
Then thanks the Doctor with a Smile.

*(Sussex Archaeological Society Library)*

personal witnesses of his present method of restoring sight. Exactly at 5 this evening the Chevalier will certainly part hence for the Castle in Brighthelmstone [Brighton[,'

He was in Lewes again a year later 'at his usual lodgings in the town'. His return was preceded by the following impressive announcement in the *Sussex Weekly Advertiser*:

'We can assure our readers that the Chevalier Taylor, Oculist, Pontificial, Imperial and Royal – namely to all the Crown'd Heads and Sovereign Princes in Europe – is now drawing towards the conclusion of his Fourth and last circuit thro' these Kingdoms, and has fixed his arrival at the White Hart in this Town for Saturday fortnight, in the evening of which all those who require his aid for defects of sight are desired to take notice. The Chevalier has been now upwards of 30 years in the greatest practice in the cure of Distemper'd Eyes of any in this age we have, and since that time has been in every Court, Kingdom, Province, State, City, and Town of the least consideration in all Europe, without exception. He is now on his return from South Wales, where from the many persons of note who recovered their sight by his hands, and the number of people he has that way made happy, he is in all places so attended that in many places his lodgings are almost inaccessible.'

Meanwhile his autobiography had appeared: *The History of the Travels and Adventures of the Chevalier Taylor, Ophthalmiator – written by Himself* in 1761 and the *Sussex Weekly Advertiser* assured that copies could be had 'on his arrival'. The book contains the famous account of the Chevalier's operations on the composers Bach and Handel, both of which were in fact unsuccessful. According to the *Spenersche Zeitung* of Leipzig for 31 July 1750, Bach died 'as an unfortunate consequence of an operation very badly performed on his eyes by a well-known English oculist'. In his *History* . . ., Taylor claimed to have been successful with Bach ('He received his sight by my hands') but more or less admitted failure with Handel ('upon drawing the curtain we found the bottom defective with a paralytic

32

disorder'). What were these failures, however, compared with the 80,000 successes which he claimed to have accomplished in 30 years! During the short stay at the White Hart in Lewes in August 1762 'his lodgings were continually crowded with persons complaining of defects of sight assembled from various parts of the county.'

Ten years later he died in a convent in Prague, blind at the last himself.


## CHARMS

The people of olden time Sussex were only too aware that the combined services of doctors, cunning folk, quacks and home remedies could be all but powerless to cure many of the conditions, ranging from plague and ague to toothache, which threatened their lives and happiness. So it made good sense to take whatever precautions they could against becoming afflicted with such conditions or diseases in the first place. Certainly, this could mean taking material precautions in the modern sense (avoiding contagion; measures of prophylactic hygiene which then could entail letting blood from the right part of the body on the right day of the month etc). But the causes of most diseases were still unknown or contentious, explained by a plethora of theories ancient and modern, and the one thing the average countryman knew for certain was that all illness was an expression of evil, attributable directly or indirectly to the Devil, witches, malign fairies, or other evil or ambiguous powers. The first line of defence against disease lay in getting the forces of good on one's side to keep evil influences at bay. This could mean deploying (taking preparations made from, burning as a fumigant, hanging from one's doors and windows) holy herbs such as St John's wort, vervain, or mugwort, regarded as especially powerful at driving away evil and its agents. Many of these were genuinely effective because they possessed real curative properties, or were good at driving 'worms' or 'snakes' from the body, or fleas, flies and lice from the body, wardrobe or house. Such precautions could also mean calling on the help of the powers of good by prayer or protective charms.

The post-medieval protestant-leaning Church increasingly frowned on the use of prayer and the help or intervention of the priest in preventing or curing disease; if the disease wasn't an ineluctable test 'sent to try one', its arrival and course weren't open to special plea-bargaining with God, Christ, or the then demoted Saints. Consequently people in a populace still imbued with the older world view and an older religion increasingly turned to the recitation of prophylactic charms, ever more distorted memories of ancient, often medieval prayers or invocations to Christ or His Saints. These were believed to be efficacious in the prevention of some particular disease, imbued with the powerful magics of religion and numerology (thrice repeated to forge a link with the Trinity, nine times because thrice three was even more powerful) and incantation. The general tendency was for charms to degenerate with time and oral transmission from initial clarity into almost total incomprehensibility.

A pocket account book used by John Skinner, a farrier of Strood Green (between Wisborough Green and Petworth), during the period 1690-1732, has been preserved. Among other items are the following:

'*A charme for a Oxe*
My Lord and my Lady went over the Sea Seven year that is past my Lord made fish my Lord made flesh my Lord made food for man and beast I charge the blader to break behinde or before in the name of God Amen.'
'*A charme for Augu and Feaver*
When Jesus saw the Cros where one his body should be crucified it be Gan to Shake the Jeues Asked what hast Ye an Augu he answered him and said whoo so ever kepes this saying in mind or writing shall neither be trobled with neather Augu or feavear. So Lord help thy servant who putteth his trust in thee Amen.'

The two charms are followed by a recipe for a remedy:

'Half a gallon of adder Spears, henbane, fetherfoy parselly sage early grass Rebwortt camamoil, cumferry, hemlock of each a handful'.

Fetherfoy is feverfew; cumferry, comfrey, and camamoil, chamomile. 'Adder spear' can be Sussex dialect for a dragonfly, but in the context of a recipe is probably the adder's tongue fern *Ophioglossum vulgatum*, principal ingredient of an 'adder's spear ointment' formerly made in Sussex and Surrey.

There is no indication as to what the remedy, or fragment of a remedy, is for, but with henbane and hemlock among its ingredients it looks decidedly deadly and may have been for external rather than internal application.

# COBWEBS

The most popular Sussex remedy for a bad cut used to be a bandage made from cobweb (for other wound cures see **Bracket Fungus, Dog, Egg, Frog, Insects, Snails, Woundworts**).

The documented history of cobweb medicine begins in antiquity, with Dioscorides, a Greek doctor who served in the army of Nero. In his *Materia Medica*, he describes how he used pads of cobweb moistened with olive oil to staunch wounds on the battlefield.

The *Materia Medica* was copied and recopied and survived the Dark Ages to become, with Celsius and Galen, one of the standard texts of English medicine during the medieval, Elizabethan and Stuart periods. We have no way of knowing whether the use of spiders' webs to staunch blood had always been practised in England since the earliest times, or was introduced in medieval to 17th century translations of Dioscorides and Celsius. Be that as it may, from the 16th-18th centuries the use of cobwebs to heal wounds was standard in both 'official' and 'folk' medicine. Thereafter it disappeared from official medical practice, but remained popular with the rural population.

In the 15th century, English soldiers at Crecy and Agincourt carried little boxes of cobweb into battle for the purpose of staunching bleeding.

In Shakespeare's *A Midsummer Night's Dream*, Bottom says 'Good Master Cobweb, if I cut my finger, I shall make bold with you'. Martin Lister in Chapter 8 of his book *British Spiders* (1678), 'Of medicaments from Spiders', included

'9. Cobwebs, tightly bound to a wound, for staunching the flow of blood; 10. The same heal open sores, congeal them, protect them from sanies [ie pus], and ward off inflammation; 11. The same for nasal haemorrhage [ie nose-bleeds] and for menstrual flow, applied internally or externally'.

Closer to home, John Goodyer, the Hampshire and West Sussex botanist, noted in his *Commentaries on Dioscorides* (1657 edition):

'The spider being wrought into one masse with a plaister, and spread upon linen, and soe layed to ye forehead or temples, doth cure the periodicall circuits of tertain agues. The cobweb of it being layed on doth staunch blood, and keeps such rotting ulcers as may break out at ye top of the skinne from inflaming.'

Spider webs remained popular in the 18th century. Here is Lawrence Sterne in *A Political Romance* (1759):

'When his Reverence cut his Finger in paring an Apple, he [Tom] went half a Mile to ask a cunning Woman what was good to staunch Blood, and returned with a Cobweb in his Breeches Pocket'.

Eleazer Albin beat cobweb with frogs' spawn and allowed the mixture to dry on a pewter plate before applying it to wounds. He writes:

'With this remedy I saved a gentleman of worth in Lincoln Inn Fields, who had bled at the nose several hours, when all applications failed which were used by two eminent surgeons'.

By this time many 'eminent surgeons' and doctors generally were beginning to view cobweb cures as dangerous folk nonsense (what happens if the web is dirty?), an attitude which was to persist into the 19th and 20th centuries. But cobwebs remained the most popular of all folk cures for wounds, their use in rural Sussex being recorded well into the late 19th and early to mid 20th centuries. Sussex author Lilian Candlin, for example, writes:

'The old established belief that a cobweb tied over a wound will stop excessive bleeding was in evidence in my childhood. I once saw a butcher at Lewes who had chopped his finger bind it up with a cobweb, dirt and all. Recently there was a report in a local paper of a man very badly cut with a piece of farm machinery arriving at hospital with a spider's web tied in the wound. The doctors admitted that had this not been done the man would have bled to death before reaching the hospital.'

The use of cobwebs to heal wounds was among the cures prescribed by old Grandmother Huggett, one of the last Sussex wise women (see under **Cunning Folk**).

And here's another account from a correspondent:

'When we were living in Heyshott, some 30 years ago, we had an old gardener who appeared for his morning coffee one day with his forefinger adorned with a dirty and gory bandage. He told me that he'd 'got himself' with the sickle and refused my first aid, saying that he'd dressed it with cobwebs and sump oil!

'During the next week, the dressing got larger and further rags were wound round it, and I became increasingly concerned. Then one day he arrived with bandage gone and a beautifully healed wound – it had been a deep one, nearly removing the nail and down to the bone, and over an inch long.

'I have never had the courage to try that one myself.'

As the perfect healing of the gardener's wound suggests, cobwebs really do possess remarkable styptic and antiseptic properties, and recent research has confirmed that Dioscorides and Grandma were right all along.

First, like cotton wool, cobweb pads provide an intricate 3-dimensional scaffolding of fibres which both absorb and aid the coagulation of blood.

Second, some of the proteins on the surface of web silk actively provoke and act as nuclei for blood coagulation.

Third, cobweb is charged with static electricity. The bacteria responsible for sepsis bear a net electric charge of the opposite sign so, as like charges repel, cobwebs repel harmful bacteria from the wound.

It is easy to see why cobwebs were the most popular of all the many rural wound cures. Cobweb cures are effective, safe, easy to remember, and spiders' webs are available all year round. Many of the other rural cures were effective too, but their ingredients were not everywhere available all year round (frogs, snails, 'woundworts' with a local distribution or short season); some were potentially risky (the lick of a dog was an effective cure, but might lead to the transmission of diseases such as rabies); and others, involving the use of woundworts, demanded a level of herbal knowledge which was not always as general in rural communities as we would sometimes like to imagine.

## Cow, horse and sheep

Our forefathers believed that the breath of large herbivores such as cows, sheep, and horses was an excellent cure for bronchial and pulmonary complaints including bronchitis, consumption, and whooping cough; particularly in a confined space – a sheep pen, cattle byre, stable or similar – where a good old 'fug' had time to accumulate.

In the Rogate region, for example, someone with whooping

cough had merely to stand under a horse and let it breathe over him, inhaling the equine's exhalations, to obtain a certain cure. Unfortunately, not just any equine would do: it had to be a skewbald for the treatment to work properly. A Chichester correspondent, Mr I.C. Faulds, recalls his father telling him that in the nearby downland village of Chilgrove, around the turn of the century, consumptives were told to go and breathe in and out deeply in the company of close-penned or huddled sheep or cows.

As recently as 1936, a Sussex shepherd was heard to recommend this cure:

'They do say that if people with consumption walk about in among the sheep in the morning when they leave the fold, it will do them a power of good. Sheep have a funny smell – not a nasty one, but a very earthy one, and they say that this is what does the consumptives good.'

## COWFOLD CHURCHWARDENS' ACCOUNTS

The Cowfold Churchwardens' Accounts for the reign of Edward IV are among the few documents that have come down to us throwing light on health, disease and medicine in Sussex before 1500. In a sense they fall beyond the scope of this book, as they belong to the ordered late medieval world with its settled medical theories and orderly rules of health, its fixed calendar of days for fasting, for eating or avoiding certain foods, or for bloodletting; days when it was advisable to take preventive precautions; and parlous days when death loomed near, rather than to the chaotic pre-modern period of competing medical theories and practices and official and folk medicines, of surgeons, doctors vying with quacks, mountebanks, charlatans, white witches, wise women and cunning men. But they are of local interest and may be worthy of inclusion because, for those who don't mind wrestling with Middle English, they make fascinating and illuminating reading.

The relevant part of the document begins with a recipe 'ffor the pestilencie to make a drynke' (see **Plague**), and goes on to give these rules for health:

'In the month of Genever [January] het es god to drynke on drawt of whet weyn [white wine] ffastyng, and vij [seven: j representing i] parlys [parlous, dangerous] dayes ther ben to be lete blod, that es ffor to say 1st day iij, v, x, xxv, xix.

'In the month of Genever [so written by mistake for Ffebrier] ette no worts [decoctions, broth] made of malowes [marsh mallow], ffor than they be parlys. Be let blode at the vayne [vein] off the thome [thumb], and ther be iiij parlys dayes – ij, iiij, xxiiij, xxvj. And in these monthe use hot mets [in the old sense of hot dishes or food, not specifically meat].

'In the monthe of Marge ette feggs [figs] and resones [raisins] and other seswet mets, and drynke swet drinks; bathe the nat thes monthe, but make las they blode [let blood] on they ryt arme en the xvij day or the last day ffor the axses and they seyt that there be iiij parlus dayes the j, xxiij, xxv, xxvj. [axes being ague, eg Chaucer in his 'Complaint of the Black Knight': "And overmore distreynd with sicknesse,/Beeside all this, he was full grievously,/For upon him he hat hot accesse/That day by day shook him piteously"]

'In the monthe off Averel be let blode on the leffte arme the x day or the xi and thou shalt not lese they sight that yer by reson: also be let blode iij dayes and thou shalt not soffer moche hed ache that yer: ette ffreych mete ffleysh, and use hot mets: and ij parleys dayes there be xx, xxv

'In the monthe off May aryse up rathe [early, eg Milton in *Lycidas* 'Bring the rathe primrose that forsaken dies] and dyny and drynke,and use hot mets: ete not no ffet [fat] of no best [beast]: be let blode on what arme thou wolle, on the iiij day,or v,or in the best day: v parlis dayes ther be – the first day iij, vj, xxv, the xxvj

'In the monthe of Juing drynke every day ffastyng a draught off water ffastyng erly and affterwarde ale or mede; ete a lytel, not ofte: thou myght be let blod thou wolle, bot ther be iiij parlous dayes – the x, xj, xxiiij, xxxix

40

'In the monthe of Julis absteyn ye ffro . . ?, for then the brayn gaderryth wormys togeder: also let not they self to blode in this monthe; viij parlus dayes there be – j, vij, xv, xiij, xij, xxv, xx [one parlous day missing or lost to fading or wear]

'In the monthe of Agoust wolle not thou to ete worts [plants] of malowes nother off cawlys [nor cabbages] and make not les they blode: vj be parlys dayes j, x, xv, xiij, xix, and xxx

'In the month of September ete rype ffryt [ripe fruit] and do the to blede and [word apparently lost or omitted from the original document] and thou wolle the xvij day; het is gode for the dropsy and for the fallyng sore. v parlus ther be – iij, vij, xiiij, xxj, xxix

'In the monthe off October het es gode to drynke must or new weyn and ffor nede thou mayste let the blode; iij parlus dayes there be iij, xviij, xxij

'In the monthe of November bathe the nat ne be nat stynted for than thy blode es gaderyd, for then het is gode to make lasse the blode of thy vaynis for than the humerys [humours] be fulle gretly multiplad; and ther be v parlus dayes j, ij, v, xj, xxviij

'In the monthe off December use hot mets, and wolle the nat then to ete worts bot gruel: and ther be v parlys dayes the vj, xiij, xxij, xxiij [fifth parlous day omitted or faded/worn away].'


## COWPATS

In the Middle Ages and until into the 18th century, rural self-help medicine made extensive use of remedies made from all manner of animal dungs (see the use of 'Goos dung' in the Sow Yallows recipe, **Livestock Remedies**). The tradition lived on into the present century. Here is 94-year old Edith Ayling talking to historian Peter Jerrome in the excellent *Petworth Society Magazine*, September 1994, about her childhood in the then remote West Sussex hamlet of Bexley Hill:

41

'Strangers brought a bit of life to the hamlet, a breath of the outside world. My brother had a boil and the old gypsy woman [who had stopped at the house] asked what was the matter with him. My mother said "He's got this terrible abscess and it's so painful". The old lady said "There's some cows in the meadow. Get the liquid from a cowpat and put it on that child's abscess and it'll be broken before he has his dinner". My mother thought it was a disgusting idea and refused to do it but my brother was in such pain that he sneaked out and did it. It worked.'

# CUCKOOS

Among the great corpus of cuckoo lore in Sussex one finds the curious belief that sufferers from lumbago will get relief by rolling on the ground at the first cuckoo call of spring; and the notion that the ashes of a roasted cuckoo would relieve pains in the stomach, fits and malaria (ague). The first cure is feasible – if unlikely to be very helpful – but the second verges on the impossible, and I cannot imagine that it was ever put into practice. Firstly, because it would surely have been more difficult to capture or kill a cuckoo than any other native bird (cuckoos are elusive and seldom seen, are not easily attracted to a food bait, unless you are very good at catching lots of hairy caterpillars and, for obvious reasons, cannot be captured when sitting on a nest). Secondly because it was considered unlucky to bring a cuckoo into the house (though I suppose one could get round this by roasting it in or over a bonfire).

For other remedies involving birds, see under **Swallow** entry, which also includes Owl Broth.

# CUNNING FOLK
## Three Portraits:

### 1. PHIL LADDS

In 1792 the humble profession of Phil Ladds was that of sow-gelder, but he gained a great reputation in Lewes and the neighbouring villages for his physic and pills, which the cottagers often preferred to those of the qualified medical men.

One day, when he was visiting Glynde, an old villager named Betsy Burgen called him into her cottage for a consultation. 'My darter,' she said, 'is troubled with two bad complaints, Mus Ladds, an' I want you to cure 'em. She's got a lying tongue an' a bad mem'ry, an' I should be glad if you could get rid of 'em for me.'

'Ah well,' replied Ladds, 'I haven't got the right stuff with me today; they are expensive pills, marm, but they'll cure your gal. They be half a crown for each one; I'll bring two when I'm around this way again. Parson may talk for everlasting to the gal an' she'll take no good on it, but one dose of mine will cure her in two minutes; if one doesn't do it, two will'.

The following week old Ladds brought the two pills, made of asafoetida or something equally nasty, and asked Betsy for the money agreed upon. When he had been paid he told the woman to summon her daughter. On the patient appearing he instructed her to chew a pill well for a minute or two, adding that it would do her no good unless she chewed it up very small.

The girl began to chew, but at once spat out the pill, crying 'Oh Mus Ladds, this is just beastly stuff you've given me; I can't swallow it nowhow in the wurreld'.

'Ah,' said Mus Ladds to the girl's mother, 'she spoke the truth that's certain, so I've cured her lyin' tongue; an't be sure she won't forget that pill, so I've cured her bad memr'y, too.'

\* \* \* \*

43

## 2. JANET STEER

In Lewes in the 1880s there was a certain Janet Steer who kept a shop in Malling Street and who was known as a wise woman, one of whose specialities was curing warts. Her method was to count the warts and then buy them from the patient for a halfpenny. People thought that she believed that if she sold her wisdom she would lose her gift, and that was why she used a method which left her financially the loser. Probably, to judge by similar cases elsewhere in England, wise women, white witches, cunning women and cunning men who held such views were after a discreet lapse of time tactfully thanked for their services with a gift of food or some other present in kind.

*   *   *   *

## 3. GRANDMOTHER HUGGETT'S CURES

The heyday of 'wise women', 'white witches', 'cunning women', and 'cunning men' was from the 16th to early-19th centuries, but wise women could still be found in many Sussex villages until the 1930s. However, they were fewer, and occupied a more modest niche in village life; no longer laying claim to extraordinary skills or a powerful magic, and confining themselves to advice on herbal cures for minor ailments.

Among the best accounts of the cures prescribed by one of the last village wise women are two articles by Eva Brotherton, entitled *Mrs Huggett's Infallible Cures* and *Grandmother's Cures*, in the late *Sussex County Magazine* during the 1930s. Comparison with other sources, such as the *Mrs Paddick* series in the *West Sussex Gazette*, also in the 1930s, confirms that the Grandmother Huggett portrayed in the following quotations is representative of the wise or cunning women – even if they were no longer, or seldom, described as such – who could still be found in many villages up until the Second World War:

> ' "Dearie me, mum, you do be bruised bad! Sit you down now while I get some o' my lily leaves pickled in brandy. Be they any good? Ah, that they be! There's nothing like

them for bruises. Draws them out wonderful."

'Old Mrs Huggett – outside whose Sussex cottage I had unfortunately slipped and fallen one frosty day – bustled away in search of her vaunted cure. Later I went home with a plaster of lily leaves adhering to my injured knee. And sure enough the charm worked, for by the next morning all traces of the bruise had nearly disappeared to the delight of my old friend, on whom I called to announce my cure.

' "There now, didn't I tell 'ee so? These old ancient things be worth a sight more than them you buy in the shops nowadays. If you were to get a cold on your chest, now, there's nothing like vinegar and whitening made into a plaster and laid on overnight. And if your throat be sore just you try flowers of sulphur swallowed dry. Ah, and if you happen to be plagued with toothache – I used to be fair tarrified of it when I were a girl – you need a nice warm poultice of poppy heads and camomile flowers boiled up together. Takes the pain away wonderful that do!" [for a very different approach to toothache, see **Gibbet**; also **Henbane**].

'I confess that I have not tried all Mrs Huggett's cures, though one or two besides the lily leaves have proved efficacious. Some are distinctly unpleasant, such as a pad of cobweb wrapped round a cut to stop the flow of blood [see **Cobweb**], or an icy-cold door-key thrust down one's back to arrest bleeding of the nose. Vinegar and brown paper or a piece of beefsteak as a remedy for black eyes are, I believe, time honoured and well-known – though Mrs Huggett did mention them, together with the 'blue bag' cure for bee and wasp stings, once universal and still better, when at hand,than anything more modern.

'She told me to apply a slice of raw potato to a wart, and that the thorn in your finger acquired while blackberrying may be drawn out by one of the leaves of the fruit moistened and left on as a plaster for an hour or two. Also of a remedy for cuts less unpleasant than cobweb: the thin membrane from inside an egg shell spread over the wound to arrest bleeding.

'Chickweed crushed and laid on as a poultice is said to act as a sedative to the pain of rheumatism, and "blanket

45

leaf" (another hedgerow plant) [this could be either the blanket leaf woundwort *Stachys lanata*, or the blanket, great or woolly mullein *Verbascum thapsus*] to make a drink which relieves whooping cough. Even now it would be hard to persuade the country-born boy or girl that dock leaves do not grow beside stinging nettles so that their coolness may be used as an antidote to the latter's burning sting.

'A curious belief still lingers in some country districts as to the efficacy of wearing a potato somewhere about the body as a cure for rheumatism. Little by little these potatoes certainly do shrivel until hard as a stone, and are then said to have absorbed and become full of the uric acid drawn from the patient's body. It is, at any rate, open to people to try this "cure" which can do no harm. Quite a number of people still have belief in it. A slice of raw potato is still used as an application for burns on the body.'

Here the Editor of the magazine comments:

'I can bear personal testimony to the efficacy of this cure. When a youngster I, one morning, upset the family coffee pot and received the contents (practically boiling) on my right leg. The result was a terrible burn from above the knee to the ankle, the scar of which I still bear as a reminder of the incident. The family nurse, an old Sussex woman, immediately set to work and with a knife scraped a number of potatoes and applied the pulp to the burn. When the doctor arrived he declared that this prompt treatment had undoubtedly saved my life, a pronouncement which I am ready to believe when I remember that the accident kept me in bed for several months.'

Other of Mrs Huggett's cures mentioned by Eva Brotherton include extract of wild campion as a good tonic, and a boiled onion for colds.

## CURSES, SPELLS AND WITCHES

Fear of witches was all too real in rural and small town Sussex from the 16th century through to the late 19th century, and anecdotes about alleged witches – Mother Digby of East Harting, Dame Garson of Duddleswell, Dame Prettylegs of Albourne, Witch Killick and Dame Neave of Crowborough, Dame Jackson of West Chiltington, and Nanny Smart of Hurstpierpoint – together with advice on how to counter their curses and spells, lingered on into the present century.

The most dreadful and dreaded power was that of bewitching, of causing sickness or even death in man or beast. When someone was stricken by a mysterious illness or when a farmer's livestock suddenly sickened and died, and witchcraft was suspected – as it usually was if the illness was mysterious and did not fall into a well-recognized category – the first step was to identify the witch who had put on the curse or spell; the second to apply counter-magic.

We have little information specific to Sussex as to how witches were identified in the early part of the great witch hysteria from the 16th to the early 18th centuries. By analogy with other counties we can presume that the suspects were subjected to rough treatment such as ducking and the search with pin or needle for insensitive devil's marks. We can get a rough idea of the fear of 'bewitching' in this period and the hysteria caused by witchcraft from the records of Sussex witchcraft trials between 1575 and the last trial in 1680.

There is only one record of the hanging of a witch in Sussex after the reign of Henry VIII. That took place in 1575, when after a trial at the Sussex Assizes held at East Grinstead, Margaret Cooper of 'Kirdeforde', wife of William Cooper, was hanged for bewitching Henry Stoner on the 1st April 'who languished until the 20th April following, when he died'.

The last recorded indictment for witchcraft in Sussex was in July 1680, when at the Assizes held at Horsham, Alice Nash was indicted for bewitching Elizabeth Slater, age 2½ years, and Anne Slater, 5½, both of whom died. In July 1654, also at Horsham, widow Jane Shoubridge of Witham was indicted for bewitching Mary Muddle, 'spinster', aged 12 years; and widow Clementine Shoubridge of Witham was severally indicted of bewitching Benjamin Caught and (presumably the same) Mary Muddle, now a 'spinster aged 13 years'. In these three cases the Grand Jury found true bills, and the indictments are endowed with the names of witnesses, but the alleged witches were acquitted by the Petty Jury and discharged. Here is a copy of one of the indictments, which makes modern legal jargon seem a paragon of clarity!:

'The Jurors for the Lord Protector of the Commonwealth of England, Scotland and Ireland, upon their oaths, doe present that Jane Shoubridge, late of Witham in the county of Sussex aforesaid, widow, the 30th day of Dec in the yeare of our Lorde one thousand six hundred fifty twoe, being a common witch and enchantress, not having God before her eyes, but being moved or seduced by the instigation of the Divell, the said 30th day of Dec of the yeare aforesaide with force and arms etc, att Witham aforesaide in the county aforesaide, certain wicked and Divelish arts called witchcraft, inchauntements, charms and sorceyres in and uppon one, Mary Muddle, spinster of the age of 12 yeares, wickedly, divelishly, feloniously, willfully and of her malice before thought did use, practyse and exercise on the said Mary Muddle then and there feloniously and of the malice before thought did bewitch and enchaunt by reason of which said wicked and divelish Arts called witchcrafts, enchauntements, Charmes and Sorceyres by her the said Jane Shoubridge in and upon the said Mary Muddle, used, practysed and exercised on the aforesaid Mary Muddle the said 30th day of Dec in the year aforesaide and divers other dayes and times as well before as afterwards att Witham aforesaide in the County aforesaide in her body was greatly wasted, consumed, pyned and harmed against the public peace and against the form of the Statute in this case made and provided . . .' And so on!

Popular belief in witches remained strong long after the 1680s, but with the learned and wealthy classes becoming increasingly sceptical, it was almost impossible to bring suspected witches to trial and the ducking or lynching of witches could bring the perpetrators themselves before courts increasingly concerned with controlling popular violence and unrest. Though rough treatment of suspected witches continued during the 18th century, people turned increasingly to roundabout ways of discovering the identity of witches responsible for particular acts of bewitchment, and countering their effects. Usually – as both the casting and lifting of spells was a specialized business – 'professional' help was sought, in the person of the local white witch, wise woman, cunning woman or cunning man, learned in cures and credited with supernatural but benevolent powers and able to provide cures or charms against illness, identify witches, operate in the witch's own territory by countering or lifting curses, spells and bewitchments, and even locate lost livestock or identify thieves.

Boys Firmin described a typical case from the 1860s. A Crowborough woman was sickening to death, and no remedy could save her until her husband, suspecting witchcraft but unsure of the witch's identity, consulted a cunning man called Oakley who lived in Tunbridge Wells. Oakley gave the husband a cupful of a liquid that had fizzed up and then went clear. He told the husband to look into it, whereupon the husband cried out exultantly: 'I see her, 'tis Witch Killick! she is the person tormenting my wife'. 'Witch' Killick was a neighbour who already had the reputation of being a witch. The cunning man then sent him home with instructions on how to counter the curse, but what they were we are, unfortunately, not told.

Home-made spells could also be used to force the witch to reveal her identity and lift the curse. Tom Reid described one such measure used when the daughter of a friend of his 'wilted and withered' after eating an orange given to her over the garden gate by a passing woman. Reid believed the counter-magic had saved the girl's life, by forcing the witch to reveal her true nature:

'First, the women of the neighbourhood should be summoned to the cottage for a chat or a cup of tea. A cauldron or pot, containing boiling water, must be hanging over the fire, and all the windows, doors and keyholes must be effectively sealed up, under cover of the women's chatter. The tips of the hair or a piece of the fingernail of all those who are present should then be flung into the boiling pot, those of the suspected witch being stealthily taken, as she would be likely to offer resistance. A witch will always scream shrilly when her nails or her hair touch boiling water whereas an ordinary mortal will show no sign at all. Should the witch not be of the party "witch noises" are to be expected outside the window.'

How it would be possible to obtain the hair and fingernails of the suspected witch is not explained.

The well-known counter-spell of the 'witch bottle' was also popular in 19th century Sussex. Mrs Latham relates how a friend of hers 'observed on a cottage hearth, a quart bottle filled with pins and was requested not to touch the bottle, as it was red hot, and if she did so she would spoil the charm.' The woman of the cottage explained that she had consulted a local wise woman about her daughter's falling [ie epileptic] fits.

'She told me that people afflicted with falling fits were bewitched and I must get as many pins as would fill a quart bottle, and let it stand close to the fire, upon the hearth, till the pins were red hot; and when that came about, they would prick the heart of the witch who had brought this affliction upon her poor girl, and who would then be glad enough to take it off.'

The effectiveness of the pins resided not just in their sharpness, but also in the fact that they were of iron, a substance traditionally believed to be of power against the forces of evil. A red hot poker was effective too: in Hastings in the 1880s a man whose wife was thought to be suffering under a spell was advised to make her sit by the hearth and to burn her wrists with a red hot poker 'to make the evil spirit fly up the chimney'. Similarly, a Crowborough tradition tells of a woman whose butter refused to 'come' no matter how hard she churned. Suspecting witchcraft her son plunged a red hot poker into the churn; there was a loud hiss or scream and soon afterwards

50

he met Dame Neave, another of Crowborough's many 'witches', hobbling down the street with a bound leg. One might also break a witch's curse by scratching her hand 'accidental like', for drawing a witch's blood has long been believed in as a means of sapping her power.

Disappointing as it may seem to some, so far as Sussex is concerned, there is no evidence to support the existence of anything like an organized witch cult with covens, black sabbaths, midnight orgies and aerial transportations. All we do find are lonely old women, living on the edge of poverty, often reduced to begging from neighbours who looked on them with contempt and resentment, and who were all too willing to blame mysterious illnesses on the evil influence of these social outcasts. The fact that they were women is only to be expected because old women and childless widows (or widows with hostile step-children) are economically and socially the most vulnerable members of small rural communities – which could be much less supportive of the no-longer-useful than we like to imagine. Often their only companions were a pet cat or toad.

It's easy to understand why in a backward, often cruel society some people – confronted by the inexplicable death of a valuable cow, or a mysterious illness in the family – should accuse others of witchcraft, and why their suspects were vulnerable, perhaps crabbed, miserable and resentful old women living alone, abandoned by or outliving their families. What is less easy to understand is why some people claimed powers of witchcraft for themselves. There are several 16th and 17th century accounts from Sussex or its adjoining regions of people claiming to be witches, not always under duress – that is at a time when witches could face the lynch mob, the ducking stool, and the gallows.

Among the main motives one may attribute to those who claimed to be witches, the desire to relieve poverty may have been the most important. For an old woman living in penury in a Tudor, Elizabethan, Stuart or Georgian village the difference between utter misery and tolerable survival may only have been a few eggs or a bag of corn. A reputation for witchcraft might, within limits, be a useful way of ensuring that her neighbours did not let her go without sustenance too often – the danger being, of course, that if a neighbour did fall mysteriously ill, things could turn very nasty. Related to the economic motive but distinct from it was the sense of power conferred on the witch by those who feared her. Again, the borderline between power feared and maleficence persecuted was a hazy one and the 'witch' herself could not always control the events which turned the community's violence against her. Perhaps an equally powerful motive was the desire for revenge against a community which she felt had abandoned her, someone to whom the usual means of revenge – the law, wealth, physical violence, social status etc – were closed.

Claiming to be, or accepting a reputation as, a witch becomes more easily comprehensible with the 19th century. The physical risks of being viewed as a witch had decreased (no lynch mobs, no gallows, though the risk of rough treatment had not wholly disappeared), while such a reputation might still bring certain small advantages in kind and a – albeit very limited – sense of power.

## THE DACRES OF HERSTMONCEUX
### Medical Expenses

The household account books of the Dacres of Herstmonceaux Castle, East Sussex, for the period 1643-9 – household here meaning everything to do with the running of the castle and estate – provide invaluable insights into the medical expenses of one of the greatest families in the land in the mid-17th century.

On only one occasion during this period of seven years did the Dacres call on the services of a physician from beyond the local community, the considerable outlay (presumably for treatment of a serious condition of one of the family, thought to be beyond the competence of local practitioners licensed or otherwise) being recorded in the following two entries.

'Deliuered unto my lord to give Dr Wilderbon's man 01 li.00.00' [ie £1]

And a few days later:

'Delieured in gould to give Dr Wilderbon's
10 li.00.00' [ie £10]

Dr Wilderbon was a celebrated physician practising at that
date in Canterbury.

This is one of the largest single outlays in the entire accounts,
and at that time amounted to at least twice the annual wage
of a day labourer.

On four occasions, the Dacres called on a local doctor,
Nehemiah Panton of Brightling. This doctor was the second
of his name to live at Brightling Place, and seems to have been
a person of some standing, sufficiently so in any case to have
been entitled to bear arms. These visits are reflected in entries
such as:

'Paid Mr Panton, Physitian, le iornaies [journeys] to Mrs
Philadelphia Lennard 3 li.'

A similar pattern emerges in the 1690s in the Duke of
Somerset's accounts for Petworth House. The local apothecary,
Mr Morris, was called in several times to treat minor ailments
– eg 'for physick and attending his Grace's children £3.3s'
– but when Lord Hertford, who died young, was very ill, Dr
Laffeaver came down from London; his fee was £32, or about
18 months wages for an estate carpenter.

A couple of points can be made here. The official practioners
were only called in to treat members of the family, not officials,
servants, or other employees in the household. However, there
are other records of nobles, rarely, and wealthy traders and
merchants, more often, calling on and paying for physicians
to treat their servants or indigent neighbours. Thus in 1732,
Richard Stapley of Hickstead Place, 'Twineham, 'Paid John
Snashall £2.14s in full for Physick and Visits to my Wife in her
sickness, and likewise paid him for the Widow Hall 10s for her
illness'. Second, though the total sums paid to Drs Wilderbon
and Panton over this seven year period – 21 livres – were
substantial in terms of the money of the time, they represent

53

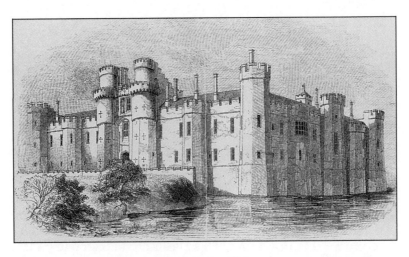

*Herstmonceux Castle, from an early 19th century woodcut. (Sussex Archaeological Society Library)*

a much lower proportion of total household expenditure than in most wealthy American or European households/ estates of the present day. As the incidence of pain and ill health was much higher, this implies a high degree of stoicism and/or a relative lack of confidence in the competence of 'physitians'.

The remaining health-related expenses of the household consist of a much larger number of entries detailing the payment of very small sums – totalling about 10 livres over seven years – to local people for medical/midwifery services and the supply of healing herbs.

In terms of volume and value the principal herb purchased by the household was samphire, which once grew abundantly along the then desolate and sparsely populated Sussex coast only a few miles to the south, and was collected on a commercial scale for sale to local communities or the London market. Thus one finds:

'Paid for 2 boshells and 1 peck of Sampher 8s.6d.'

It was used as a pickle and was also eaten as an anti-scorbutic. Another anti-scorbutic was 'Scurvie Grass', also harvested along the Sussex coast. (See **Scurvy, Scurvy grass**).

'Paid for scurvie grass for a drink for Mr Wood etc 02s.06d. Paid Tye for one jornaye from Bourne [Eastbourne] with the said scurvie grass 01s.00d.

Such entries suggest that the Dacres at least were aware that the current physicians' treatment for scurvy, involving the application of sulphuric acid, was expensive, ineffective and harmful, and that the condition was better treated by herbal or dietary means.

Several other entries refer to the purchase of herbs, for example:

'Paid for 2 li [pounds] prunes and 2d worth of worm seeds for my lords daughters 06d' [worm seeds, the seeds of the treacle mustard, were a popular vermifuge, see **Wormwood**].
    'Paid Widdow Leuis for gathering herbs 2 daies 06d. Paid a maiden for gathering herbs for my 2 young mistresses 02d'

There are also several entries detailing sums paid to local people for 'bleeding' members of the household or farm stock:

'Paid my lord beneuolence for letting blood sick folkes 10s. Paid Mr Waters for letting T. Christians blood 01s. Paid for bleeding the Kiene [cows] and young cattle and 2 men that did helpe 05s'

In ordinary cases of childbirth the attendance of a midwife was all that was thought necessary and even when a person occupying a position of importance like Lady Dacre was confined of her first child no medical assistance seems to have been sought for. The accounts for the week in which Philadelphia was born make no mention of any doctor being called in, but show that 'my Lord' gave away 'beneuolences' as follows:

'Paid my Lords beneuolence to Widdow Craddock the

55

midwife of Battle 05 li 00 00. Paid Elizabeth Squib the laundry maid 00.10.00. Paid to John Furbeck the coachman 00.5s.00. Paid John Blunden the Postilion 00.05.00'

Elizabeth Squib's occupation sufficiently explains the reason she might be considered to have a claim on 'my lords beneuolence', and if the 'beneuolences' were given to the stable men in connection with the child's birth, as was probably the case, it was no doubt to reward them for some special trouble they encountered in fetching the midwife and her assistants to the castle. The Sussex roads, always terrible in winter, were especially bad the January of Philadelphia's birth; being, as Francis Dacre said in a letter to Lord Grey, written to excuse him attendance at the House of Lords, 'extremely clogged by a very deep snow'.

Staying at the castle at the time of Lady Dacre's confinement were 'ye nurse, the midwife, Glid's wife, and diuers attendants, besides their husbands'. From other mentions in the accounts, it appears that Glid's wife was a local wise woman whose medical skills were sought for minor ailments and operations. Within six months of the child's birth, Glid's wife was back at the Castle:

'Paid to Glid's wife for cutting Mrs [sic] Philadelphia's tongue 02s 6d'


## A DOCTOR ADVERTISES

The card reproduced here is a trade card of a kind which would not be allowed nowadays, although, as the British Museum has a large collection they must have been quite usual at the period.

Mr George Dixon was a son of the curate in charge of Sullington. He rented West Chiltington Rectory and was the uncle of Mr Frederick Dixon who practised at Worthing, founded the dispensary there and was the author of the well-known work *The geology and Fossils of the Tertiary and Cretaceous Formations of Sussex*, published posthumously in 1850.

AT THE SOLICITATION OF SEVERAL RESPECTABLE FAMILIES,

# Mr. GEORGE DIXON

PROPOSES

## To Attend PATIENTS upon the following Terms :

### ( M E D I C I N E S   I N C L U D E D ).

*Within the Diſtance of FOUR Miles,*

Attendance every Day, . . . . . . . . TWO GUINEAS a Week,
Three Times a Week, . . . . . . . . . ONE GUINEA,
Single Visits . . . . . . . . . . . . . . HALF-A-GUINEA,
Advice at Home, Mondays, Wednesdays, and Fridays, from Nine
'till Twelve, . . . . . . . . . . . SEVEN SHILLINGS each Time.

*Within the Diſtance of SIX Miles,*
Each Visit, . . . . . . HALF-A-GUINEA.

*To TEN Miles,*
Each Visit, . , . . . . . . ONE GUINEA.

Chiltington Parsonage, near Storrington, Jan. 6, 1800.

SORRELL, PRINTER, 86, BARTHOLOMEW CLOSE.

---

*A doctor advertises — Mr Dixon's card. (Sussex Archaeological Society Library)*

Mr George Dixon was the inventor of Dixon's Pills, a popular proprietary remedy in the early 19th century.

There are a couple of points of interest here. First, at the start of the 19th century, professional medical attention was still accessible on a regular basis to no more than 5-10% of the Sussex population earnings, say, more than £100 pa (nobility and gentry, wealthier clergy, professionals and tradesmen). Persons earning £15-£100 pa (for example village schoolmaster £15-£30, skilled carpenters £15-£35) might be able to afford a doctor in a crisis, but not regular or prolonged attention or treatment. The great majority of the population earning £5-£15 pa couldn't afford doctors, full stop – though they might have some access to treatment under the Poor Law (ranging from negligible to generous from parish to parish). Thus it had been for more than 200 years, and thus things were to remain for another 120 years.

Second, the doubling of the fee for visits to patients living more than six miles from West Chiltington underlines the extent to which access to medical care depended on considerations of geography. Most doctors were based in towns and in large prosperous villages, mainly along the coast and scarp-foot zone north of the Downs. Because of the notoriously poor state of the Sussex 'roads' and tracks – the worst in Britain south of the Peak and east of Dartmoor – visits to outlying villages, hamlets and farms were time-consuming and next to impossible in bad winter weather: and were charged accordingly. Wealthy people in outlying parts, and notably in the High Weald, had to live with, and adapt to, the reality that even though they could afford the services of a doctor, he might not get through in time (allowing at least three hours for a servant to get through to the doctor, three or four hours for the doctor's journey, double or quadruple that if the doctor was out or the ways were impassable with mud or snow). Less wealthy people had to adapt to the reality that the doctor might not get through in time *and* that his fee would include a large, often prohibitive, call-out charge. Small wonder, then, that in remoter areas of Sussex people at every level of society took a keen interest in traditional self-help rural medicine, and that cunning folk with recognized healing skills were thick on the ground and valued members of the local community.

## Dogs healing and dogs mad

Dog and cow saliva are rich in recently-discovered chemical factors known as Transforming Growth Factors (TGFs), which possess a remarkable ability to induce cell division (ie multiplication) and differentiation. These factors are present in human saliva, but only as insignificant traces.

Recent research has shown that TGF-rich extracts prepared from canine and bovine saliva accelerate wound healing in human accident and burn victims. A result which helps explain why dogs lick their wounds so assiduously (they are doing more than just cleaning the wound); and why a friendly healing lick from a dog is a traditional treatment for cuts, wounds and burns, recorded in cultures as far removed in time and space as Ancient Egypt, Ancient Greece, 15th-19th century Sussex – Charlotte Smith, the great 18th century Sussex poet and novelist, writes of country people in Sussex getting dogs to lick their wounds – and 20th century Fiji.

Perhaps, however, I should recount a cautionary tale. Sir Alexander Fleming, discoverer of penicillin, discusses the case of a man who allowed an apparently healthy dog to lick a gash on his leg, in the well-founded belief that a lick from a dog accelerates healing. The wound healed perfectly. But some time later, the man died the terrible death reserved for those who contract rabies.

The risk of dying from a healing lick was not negligible; rabies was a terrifying reality of English life until the late 19th century. So it is no surprise that a great many cures were devoted to treating the bites of 'madde dogges' – whether the victim was human, a horse, pig, sheep or cow (all too valuable to be allowed to die without a fight) – though it is doubtful if any of the remedies could have had an effect on what was virtually an incurable, and almost invariably fatal, disease.

Here is a Sussex example noted down in the account books of Timothy Butt of Tillington, c1765-1800:

'For a Bite of a Mad Dogg for cattle etc. Take bittaney, Night Shade, lungeworte, Arbegrass, Read Sage, Box, Primrose Root, Daisey Roots, Alleuffs, Madder, half an ounce of Anniseed, Carraway seed, Coming seed, Callender seed, in all half an oz, when mingled and beat to a powder. Screed the Arbs [herbs] very small, take 3 spoonsfull and put it to powder for one bulloch or a Hogg and put it all into a pint of Milk'

And here is a 16th century procedure 'To know the bite of a madde dogge':

'If the same day that you have beene bitten of a dogge (which you doubt to have been madde) you put upon the biting an old walnut well braied [roasted, from old English braedan = to roast], and after take it away, and caste it to a hungry cocke or hen, if the same eating it die not, it is a sign that the dogge which did bite you was not madde, but if it die, then it is a sign that he was madde and therefore the same must be looked into as is meete within three daies.'

## EARNINGS AND THE AFFORDABILITY OF MEDICINE

The earnings of the wealthiest section of the population in 17th and 18th century Sussex (the aristocracy, large landowners, prosperous farmers on the coastal plain and Downs; furriers, ironmasters, some surgeons, lawyers, mercers etc) were comparable with those of their counterparts elsewhere in lowland east, central and southern England. However, they comprised a smaller proportion of the population, and earnings of small farmers, agricultural labourers, small traders and artisans, village curates and schoolmasters etc were much lower than in, say, Hampshire, Somerset, the Thames Valley, or East Anglia.

There were foci of wealth: the great estates, large farms on the plain and Downs, some lucrative export trades, and the Wealden iron industry before its decline, but much of Sussex was still remote and isolated behind the barrier of the Weald with its near-impassable tracks, and this exerted a strong downward pressure on the earnings and spending power of the poorer members of the community. Their isolation and limited mobility were important factors, others were the almost total absence of competition from early industries, for example textiles, and the lack of opportunities to supplement income from smaller scale rural occupations such as pin-making, copperas-boiling, starch-making, and lace, ribbon, button, thread, and cloth-making, which were directly or indirectly pushing up earnings in many other rural areas.

In the Weald, which made up some two-thirds of Sussex, the great majority of the population lived in households with earnings below, often substantially below, £70 per annum. There were almost no £200-a-year farms, few £100 farms; cottagers and labourers had incomes of no more than £5-£20 pa even when bounties, outworking, children in service etc are taken into account; small artisans, village schoolmasters etc were mainly in the £15-£45 range. But the wealthy *were* wealthy: with a scattering of gentry, ironmasters, furriers etc in the £500-£800 + range, and a slightly broader scattering of mercers, butchers, millers, publicans and so on in the £70 + range (though proportionally fewer than in most lowland counties because there was less wealth to trickle down, and less spending power around).

This is reflected in a paucity of surgeons and apothecaries and in their relatively low earnings, these mainly in the comfortable but far from glorious £100-£300/400 range. Though there is evidence that some physicians charged slightly lower fees than their counterparts in more prosperous regions, their principal strategy was to keep fees high and to have a large territory, treating a relatively small number of wealthy patrons or tolerably comfortable clients in several or many parishes. Their fees were supplemented by Poor Law earnings which were generally meagre in impoverished areas because the resources available for relief were limited. The size of physicians' territories, hence the success of this strategy, was limited both by competition, and the atrocious state of the tracks and fear of footpads.

Moving into the southern third of Sussex, the earnings triangle takes on a healthier profile with more prosperous farmers whose farms were worth £200-£500, even £1,000 + a year, wealthier curates, professionals and 'tradesmen' (blacksmiths, butchers, coopers, cordwainers, cutlers, glovers, haberdashers, innkeepers, millers, tanners etc) with earnings of £70-£700 pa; and better, though still low, earnings for small tradesmen, schoolmasters etc. Nonetheless, the majority of the population was left living in households with earnings of less than £70 pa.

The greater density of people who could afford medicine is reflected in a greater density of, and higher earnings for, physicians. Their territories were smaller, and their earnings mainly in the range £100-£700 pa, perhaps more if they were fashionable or ran successful smallpox inoculation clinics.

Single visits from physicians cost half a guinea, a guinea and upwards. Assuming that household could assign no more than 5-15% of its annual income to medical expenses (just 5% if the family was poor and hard-pressed by competing expenses), it is clear that the many people in Sussex living in households earning less than £20-£30 pa simply didn't have access to licensed medicine, except under Poor Law provisions. Above this figure, people might be able to afford occasional visits or short courses of treatment, but only the small proportion of the population in households with incomes above, say £300 pa could afford the services of a 'family doctor' in the fullest sense of the words, or sustained treatment during a serious, long illness.

From 1800 onwards average earnings in Sussex rose slightly faster than doctors' fees, and faster than elsewhere in England because there was a lot of catching up as the county was opened up by better roads and the railways. But this was only on average, as there was great local variation, with some areas of the High Weald remaining notably poor; and some occupations, for example agricultural labourers, lagging behind.

So in general the proportion of people who could afford at least occasional medical treatment increased. But as late as the 1890s-1930s many people were still too poor to afford the (by now, on balance, beneficial!) services of a doctor, except under the Poor Law or through the charity of a neighbour. And most of those who could afford some treatment lived in fear of the prolonged serious illness which would confront them with a no-win choice between impotent suffering and unpayable medical bills.

## EASTER BUNS

The special food of Good Friday was and is the hot cross bun. There was at one time in Sussex a firm belief that these buns, and also any loaves of bread baked on this day, had powerful curative and protective powers. Small loaves baked on Good Friday were given to children to keep all year. In many cottages and farmhouses, a hot cross bun would be kept all year for luck, hung up by the hearth, or from a roof beam in the kitchen, or stored in a tin; it was said to protect the house from fire and witches, and a few crumbs grated from it or a slice from the outside mashed with milk were sometimes taken as a medicine for all manner of ailments or applied to cuts, wounds, abscesses, whitlows, etc.

Here, for example, is Frederick Ernest Sawyer writing about 'Sussex Folk Lore and Customs Associated with the Seasons' in the *Sussex Archaeological Collections* some 70 years ago:

'GOOD FRIDAY. It is almost a religious duty in Sussex to eat buns on this day, which buns are kept until the next Good Friday for luck, being preserved in tin boxes. A Brighton baker has informed me, that a local undertaker (lately deceased) always kept a cross bun by him, replacing the old by a new one each Good Friday. Mr Henderson says they have been hung up in Sussex cottages, and when illness broke out in the family, a fragment is cut off, powdered, and *given as a medicine!* [Sawyer's emphasis] I am also informed (by Mr John Sawyer) that to keep a cross bun in the house is thought by some Sussex folks a preservative against fire.'

Opinion differed as to whether the bun or loaf should be baked extra hard, or baked soft and allowed to become mouldy. The hard-baked bun or loaf would have kept well all year round, but would have possessed only magical or psychological rather than direct physical, curative powers. The softer bun or loaf allowed to go mouldy would have kept less well, but possessed real curative virtues (see **Moulds**).


# Eggs

'Nothing better for cuts and bruises than the petals of the Madonna lily, pickled in brandy and laid on as a skin, which adheres to the injured part, healing it and keeping it clean at the same time; as does the thin membrane from the inside of an egg-shell . . .' (Eva Brotherton, writing on the cures of Grand-mother Huggett in 1939 – see also under **Cunning Folk**).


# ELECAMPANE

A native of Central Asia, elecampane was brought to Britain as a medicinal plant before or during the Middle Ages and widely grown in Sussex physic and cottage gardens until the late 18th century. It is no longer a popular garden plant, but can still be found wild at a few localities scattered across Sussex, where it is an escapee from or relict of past cultivation. Deep-rooted and enduring, elecampane will long outlast home or garden. The *Sussex Plant Atlas* records it at six sites in West Sussex and ten in East Sussex.

De l'Obel and Gerard in the 16th century knew it not only as one of the most valuable plants of the physic garden, but also much as we know it – in meadowbank, downland and, long escaped, long established, in old orchards.

It is an impressive plant about three ft high with enormous dock-like leaves up to two ft long by nine inches wide; these leaves were sometimes used as bandages for wounds, though this seems to have been a very secondary use. The light yellow flowers, about two inches wide, resemble those of a marigold, but with narrower petals. It is a close relative of two natives: the golden samphire, which grows sparingly along the Sussex coast, and was used against scurvy (see **Charlatans: Dr Flugger** and **Dacres Family**); and ploughman's spikenard, that tall, solitary plant of the South Downs which may have been used in plague cures, see **Plague**.

*The Englishman's Doctor* 1608, Sir John Harington's translation of the medieval *Regimen Sanitatis Salernitatum*, laid out its virtues in the following terms:

'Ellecompane strengthens each inward part,/A little looseness is thereby provoken/It swayeth griefe of minde, and cheeres the heart,/Allaieth wrath/And makes a man

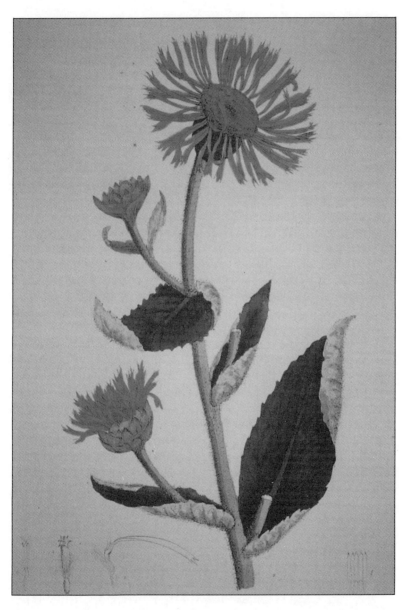

*Elecampane from an illustration in* Flora Medica, *1829. (Royal Botanic Gardens, Kew)*

faire spoken:/And drunk with Rue in wine, it doth impart/Great help to those that have their bellies broken.'

Leaving out the traditional use against snakes and snake-bite, John Pechey (*Compleat Herbal*, 1694) summarized the virtues of elecampane, or rather of the sweet-smelling and aromatic t ng but also bitter roots:

'The fresh Root being candied, or dried, and powder'd, mix'd with Honey or Sugar, is very good in a Difficulty of Breathing, an Asthma, and an old Cough. Being taken after supper, it helps Concoction. It is also commended as an excellent preservative against the Plague. Being taken in the Morning, it forces Urine and the Courses. Half a pint of White Wine wherein the Slic'd Roots have been infused three days, taken in the morning fasting, cures the Green-sickness. A Decoction of the Root, taken inwardly, or outwardly applied, is commended by some for Convulsions, Contusions, and the Hip-Gout. The Roots boiled in Wine, or the fresh Juice infus'd in it, and drunk, kills and expels Worms. Wine that is every where prepar'd with this Root in *Germany*, and often drunk, wonderfully quickens the sight.'

Though elecampane was thus deemed to have countless virtues, it is most often mentioned in surviving Sussex sources in the form of an infusion or syrup, as an ingredient in remedies for asthma, bronchitis, cold, consumption (TB), coughs, pneumonia, and whooping cough. Here is a typical recipe from Edward Austin's *Approved Medicines and Receipts* (Burwash, 1701):

'A scirrop for a Consumtick Coff. Take one part of white wine and one oz of lickquorish powder, and 1 oz of the powder of Arnica seeds, and 1 oz of sugar candy, and ½ an egg shell of the powder of allicampane and a Quarter of a lb of Treacle and 8 figgs slitt and stoned; put all these into ye white wine in a pewter dish, then leave the dish and set it in some charcoal and make it Boyle very softly, and as it boyles there will arise a Dew upon ye dish which you must wipe off, and after the Dew hath done rising take it off, and put it into a Gallypot for your use and take it night and morning. The same is said to be a certain cure. *Probatum Est.*'

Other sources mention 'allicompane' boiled with mallory in honey for consumption.

Recent research has shown that the active bitter principles of elecompane root is such a powerful antiseptic and bacteriocide that a few drops at a dilution of one part in 10,000 kills most ordinary bacterial organisms – and is particularly destructive of the tuberculosis bacterium responsible for consumption. So infusions and syrups of elecampane would undoubtedly have been effective against bronchial and pulmonary complaints either caused by, or likely to be complicated by, bacterial infections, such as bronchitis, persistent colds, consumption, pneumonia, and whooping cough, though less effective against viral infections such as primary colds and 'flu.

Among elecampane's dialect names in Sussex were scabwort, elf dock and horseheal, the latter a reminder that the plant was also a notable horse medicine – though its original use as a horse-heal seems, from the references to it in early English sources, to have been based on a misidentification of the Latin *Inula*, elecampane, with *hinnulus*, a young horse.

Elecampane was also used as a vegetable fly-paper, one of two in common use in 15th-18th century England. In *An Arrangement of British Plants* (7th edition, 1830), William Withering mentions that the glutinous spring leaves of the alder were sometimes strewn on floors in Hampshire and Sussex farmhouses to catch insect pests; and that the sticky, enticingly-scented roots of elecampane were hung by doors and windows to catch flies.

# FITS, A Charm For

K.A. Esdaile (*Sussex Notes and Queries* Vol. 9, 1942) writes:

'The following story was told me in 1929 by an old inhabitant of West Hoathly. The subject of the experience is a youngish woman still living in the cottage which is the scene of the story. I have altered a name, but the facts are odd enough to deserve record as taking place this century within 34 miles of London.

'Mrs Pellatt had a beautiful baby, "a lovely girl she war," and all went well till the child was two years old when, seated on a neighbour's lap at the tea table, she had a fit. The fits went on for months, and Mrs Pellatt was in despair till she remembered a cure for fits which she had heard of as a girl, and she determined to try it.

' "You must get 7 threepenny bits from 7 strange men, not saying who you are or what you want them for, and put them in a bag and tie them secretly round the child's neck, never letting them leave her, and the fits will die away."

'It took her a long time to collect the threepenny bits, but eventually she got them, put them in a bag and tied them round the child's neck. Sure enough, the fits got better and in a year or two the child was well enough to go to school. She got no worse, and nothing happened until another child saw the bag round her neck and began to "tarrify" her, the spell of secrecy was broken, and the fits returned.'

For other cures for fits, see **Cuckoo, Swallow Water**, and **Walnuts**.

# FLEAS, FLEABANE AND FLEAWORT

There was no getting away from fleas in days gone by. When parts of old Whitehall Palace were exposed during alterations

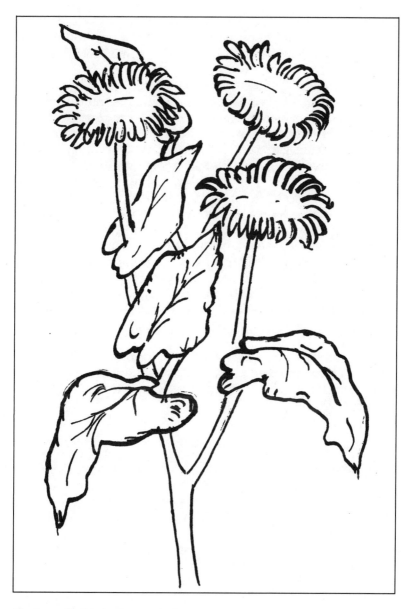

*Fleabane (Pulicaria dysenterica)*

to the Treasury in 1962 a wardrobe of Henry VIII's clothes was exposed for the first time since the 16th century. Among the royal clothes were tens of thousands of mummified Tudor fleas. Like death, fleas gave no indemnity to kings.

Until the early 19th century, Englishmen and women, rich and poor alike, were infested with and tormented by fleas, which isn't so very surprising. Houses, even or particularly the great houses and palaces of the aristocracy, were inadequately heated. So from late September to early June people of all conditions went unwashed and wore multiple layers of clothing: a combination providing optimum conditions for fleas and lice. As the clothes themselves were made of materials such as wool and fur easily damaged by frequent washing in crude detergents, they were washed infrequently, if at all, which further favoured the survival of fleas, lice, and their resting stages. The retreat of the flea from the bodies and houses of the English only began in the 19th century with the arrival of cosier heating – so that people could wash more and wear fewer clothes indoors – and cheap cotton clothes and sheets which could be washed more often and/or replaced more frequently.

The agonies which fleas inflicted on locals and travellers in Sussex in times past are vividly reflected in this passage from John Taylor's poem 'A Discovery by Sea from London to Salisbury, in the year 1623'

'A Town called Goreing stood neare two miles wide,
To which we went and had our want supplide:
There we relieued ourselves (with good compassion)
With meat and lodging of the homely fashion.
To bed we went in hope of rest and ease
But all beleaguered with an host of fleas:
Who in their fury nip'd and skip'd so hotly
That all our skins were almost turn'd to motley.
The bloudy fight endur'd at least six houres
When we (opprest with their encreasing powers)
Were glad to yield the honour of the day
Unto our foes, and rise and runne away . . .'

According to a 19th century writer in the *Collections of the Sussex Archaeological Society*:

'the First of March was notable in Sussex for its peculiar association with fleas. Everyone apparently agreed that on this particular date the creatures woke up and began hopping about, and that this was therefore the moment to get rid of them, but the suggested methods differed sharply.'

In West Sussex the dominant belief was expressed in the rhyme: 'If from fleas you would be free,/Let all your doors and windows open be'.

Consequently, people would get up before dawn to fling their doors and windows open with the cry 'Welcome, March!'; sometimes also the children would be given brushes and told to sweep all dirt away from the thresholds and window sills. But some people, particularly in the east of the county, recommended the opposite procedure, with the verse:

'If from fleas you would be free,
On the First of March let your windows closed be.'

The custom is still sometimes remembered, though presumably not acted on. For instance, an informant at Littlington in East Sussex said in 1965 that the reason the windows were always kept shut in March was that it was believed the winds blew the fleas out of the thatch. The blustery winds of March are notorious; indeed, as the prevailing direction of the wind is from the west, I have heard the sarcastic comment that if the people of West Sussex are opening their windows on this date, it is only natural that those of the East should close theirs. Moreover, the people of Arundel had at one time a method of their own – on this date they went and shook themselves on Arundel Bridge, in the belief that this would keep them free of fleas for the rest of the year.

But fleas did not have it all their own way and Sussex people were not everywhere as helpless in their presence as travellers' tales and this picturesque but ineffectual response would suggest. In rural Sussex there were four great strewing herbs of use against fleas: fleabane, mugwort, wormwood and rue. All four are violently aromatic. All have stems, leaves, or flowers loaded with fragrant insecticidal chemicals. And all four, strewn on the floor or burned to give a fumigatory smoke, will drive fleas from the house. If rural labourers, husbandmen, yeoman, local clergy, minor gentry, and their families were less flea and lice-infested than the notoriously verminous urban poor, artistocracy and royalty it was partly because they were able and willing to exploit this traditional rural lore.

The name fleabane is self-explanatory. In Old English, *banes* were outright poisoning plants (cf Old Norse *bani*, Old German *banu*, destruction, death).

A single bite of cowbane (*Cicuta virosa*, a sister plant of hemlock) sends a cow into fatal convulsions. Horsebane (the dead tongue, *Oenanthe crocata*), sowbane (*Chiropodium rubrum*) and henbane (the deadly nightshade relative *Hyoscyamus niger*) will kill horses, sows, hens, and most other creatures. Medieval wolf hunters used the deadly convulsant juice of the wolfbane, *Aconitum*, to tip their arrows and poison baits. And fleabane, true to its name, kills fleas.

Several 'fleabanes' 'fleaweeds' and 'fleaworts' grow wild in Sussex, but *Pulicaria dysenterica*, the common fleabane or 'daisy' of damp grassland and damp, marshy roadsides was the one most used to fumigate wardrobes and rooms. It is a pretty little plant with furry wrinkled leaves, bright yellow flowers which scarcely peep above the level of the grass and, especially if you crush the leaves, a faint tell-tale odour of cats, carbolic and chrysanthemums.

The odour of chrysanthemums is the give-away. The well-known insecticide *pyrethrum* is made from the dried powdered flower heads of the insect plant *Chrysanthemum cinerarii*, possibly indigenous to south-east Europe and the Middle East, but now cultivated around the world. Fleabanes are chrysanthemum-relatives and also contain pyrethrums. So when Sussex housewives burned fleabanes to fumigate wardrobes and bedrooms, clouds of flea-killing pyrethrums filled the house.

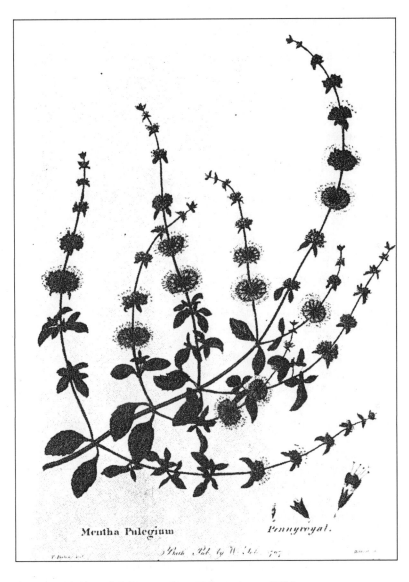

Meutha Pulegium

Pennyroyal.

*Pennyroyal from Sole's* Menthae Britannicae, *1798*

Rue, one of the great flea-killing plants of antiquity, was brought to Britain by the Romans. From the Middle Ages onwards it was grown in every Sussex physic garden and in many cottage gardens, and judges at the East Grinstead Quarter Sessions or the Lewes Assizes wore rue inside their clothes as a protection against fleas, lice, and the dreaded 'prisoner's revenge' of gaol fever (probably typhus, transmitted by lice).

An Elizabethan verse records some of the virtues, real and imaginary, for which rue was famed:

> 'Rue maketh chaste and eke preserveth sight,
> Unfuseth wit, and fleas doth put to flight.'

Mugwort (*Artemisia vulgaris*), is a common native (see **Wormwood**), and its fellow wormwood absinthe (*Artemisia absinthum*), a Bronze Age to Roman introducee best known as the active ingredient of the notorious absinthe. Both contain in all their parts some 40 insecticidal oils and alkaloids. Sussex farmers wore wormwood in their clothes to kill fleas and lice. Their wives put wormwood in wardrobes or closets to drive away clothes moths, fleas and flies (an Old French name for wormwood is *garde-robe*) and scattered wormwood on floors, following the advice given by the East Hoathly, East Sussex, agriculturist Thomas Tusser in his widely read *Five Hundred Pointes of Good Husbandrie* (1573 edition):

> 'While wormwood hath seed, get a bundle or twain,
> To save against March, to make flea to refrain,
> Where chamber is swept, and wormwood is strewn,
> No flea, for his life, dare abide to be known.'

Other Sussex flea plants were bog myrtle or gale – locally known as flea-weed – a sweetly resinous shrub formerly common on the vast Sussex Marshes, and incorporated into bedstraw to deter fleas; pennyroyal, the *pulegium* or flea plant of Dioscorides, formerly grown in cottage gardens as a cure-all and flea-deterring bedstraw; lady's bedstraw (*Galium verum*, locally flea-weed or fleawort), another sweetly-scented flea-killing plant widely used as a bedstraw; and water pepper, *Polygonum hydropiper*, used for sores, ulcers, swellings, toothache, jaundice, and as a flea-repelling bedstraw. This gave rise to the Sussex dialect name Arsesmart – widely used until the advent of the politer botanists of the 19th century – 'because if it touch the taile or other bare skinne, it maketh it smart, as often it doth, being laid unto the bed greene to kill fleas'.

A final point. Starlings weave large quantities of fleabane or lady's bedstraw into their reusable and frequently reused, hence potentially verminous nests, presumably to repel ticks, lice and fleas.


# FROGS

The aquatic South African clawed frog, *Xenopus laevis*, like the white mouse and the fruit fly, is one of those animals that could have been made with laboratories in mind. It is popular among scientists mainly because of its robust health and large eggs, for which many experimental procedures have been designed. Xenopus frogs are easy to use. Just cut one open, take out the eggs, seal it up and pop it back into its tank of water. To molecular and developmental biologists, Xenopus is an everyday part of life, like a laboratory bench or bunsen burner.

Looked at in a new way, the mundane frog becomes extraordinary. Some time ago, Dr Michael Zasloff of California University asked himself how frogs that had recently been cut open managed to avoid fatal infections when they swam around in not very clean water teeming with hungry microbes. His curiosity paid off. After a long investigation, he isolated some previously unknown anti-bacterial and antifungal substances to which he gave the name *maganins*, from the Hebrew word for shield.

Maganins are peptides manufactured by special glands in the skins of Xenopus and many other frogs, including the common English species. Peptides are made up of amino acids, as in proteins, but whereas proteins are long (at least 250 amino acids) peptides are short. The maganins isolated by Zasloff turned out to be 21-29 amino acids long, which makes them the same sort of size as hormones.

Establishing the existence of maganins opened up a whole new set of questions, many of which have yet to be answered. It is not yet clear how many types a frog has, but there seem to be at least a dozen. Each type of maganin seems to work against a slightly different range of cells and the whole family provides frogs with a protective shield against protozoa and fungi as well as bacteria. They work by making cells burst, but the mechanism by which they do so is a mystery.

I need scarcely point out the life-saving medical possibilities opened up by these newly-discovered chemicals. They may have a role in treating patients with bad wounds or burns. They might help to kill off the bacteria which infest the lungs of sufferers from cystic fibrosis. And so on.

Such uses of maganins may not be new, though, for frogs are popular ingredients of traditional remedies all around the world.

According to the ancients, frogs collected at full moon and taken internally were a good remedy for consumption (TB). The swallowing of live frogs to cure consumption was still common in Sussex 200 years ago, and there are records from as recently as the late 19th and early 20th centuries, for example, this account from the *Sussex County Magazine*, 1928:

'Chatting one day with an East Sussex policeman, he told me that when stationed in the Mayfield district he knew a resident who believed he was suffering from, or was becoming afflicted with, that malady [consumption]. Having heard of someone in the locality who had been cured of the complaint by swallowing frogs, he determined to try the remedy himself. He did so with what he believed to be great success. The constable said it was no fairy tale, as he himself had caught some young frogs for the gentleman and saw him swallow them. I met the old policeman a few years ago. He is now retired. He told me that the gentleman was now dead, but he had lived to be 80 years of age.'

It has been shown in the test tube that maganins from frog skin kill TB bacteria, so it may well be that swallowing live frogs provided at least some sort of cure for consumption. A much more convincing example is the old Sussex custom, recorded by Andrew Borde of Pevensey in the 16th century and practised in rural Sussex until the early 19th century, of strapping a live frog to a wound to help it heal without infection/festering. Since adrenalin causes the glands in the frog's skin to secrete maganins and being strapped to an invalid (or being swallowed alive, for that matter) must cause a frog plenty of stress, the frog must be pumping out maganins like mad – straight on to the wound. In times past a cure by frog would have looked like magic – now it looks like maganins.

For other cures for wounds, see **Bracket Fungus, Cobweb, Dog, Elecampane, Egg, Moulds, Snails, Woundworts;** for other cures for consumption, see **Cow, Elecampane, Mice, Snails, Wormwood** and under **Swallow**, Owl broth.


# GIBBET

Gibbets, or the corpses hanging thereon, were widely believed to possess remarkable curative virtues; and none more so than that known as 'Jacob's Post' on Ditchling Common.

The circumstances which led to the erection of this gibbet are described by John Stapley of Hickstead Place, Twineham, in a diary entry dated 26 May 1734:

'Jacob Harris, a Jew pedlar by trade, and travelling the country with his wares, having murdered at Ditchling Common, one Miles, his wife, and maid, and then plundered the house, was captured at Turner's Hill by John Oliver and his man, and committed by Mr S. Sergesson, before whom he was taken, to Horsham Gaol. Having been found guilty of the offence at the assizes, and condemned to die, he was hung at Horsham, August 31st, and his body afterwards removed to Ditchling Common to be hung on a gibbet near to the house in which the murder was committed, the 2nd day of September. Many went to see him hanging; and Mr Healey preached an impressive sermon upon it the Sunday following.'

Its subsequent history was summarized by the Revd Edward Turner in 1866:

'About five or, perhaps, six feet of this gibbet still remains above the surface of the soil in which it is fixed. All gibbets are imagined to possess a power of enchantment – some being found to be a remedy for, or preservative against, one kind of disorder, and some another. This at Ditchling Common is supposed by the inhabitants of the surrounding district to possess a peculiar preventive virtue against aching teeth, a small piece of it carried in the pocket being an effectual remedy against that racking disorder. Instances are quoted of its complete efficacy in such cases, parties being referred to who have tried the remedy for years with unfailing success. Whether they might not have been as free from pain in the teeth if they had not adopted this charm, is a point which it would be difficult now to decide. An excellent old lady, and an aunt of my mother, who lived in her single, married, and afterwards widowed state, for upwards of 80 years, at no great distance from this post, had so much faith in it that she was accustomed to expatiate largely on its efficacy, and the many instances of good she herself had known to be derived from it. And she used most amusingly to declare, that nothing should induce her to be without a piece of the far-famed gibbet in her pocket, though she had long ceased to have a tooth remaining in her jaws.
'The part of the Common on which the remaining part of this gibbet stands, and the houses about it, are still commonly called from this circumstance 'Jacob's Post.'

Slivers of wood from the gibbet were also believed to be an effective charm against evil spirits and fits. William Albery, the Horsham historian, quoted an old inhabitant of Ditchling who said: 'People come from moiles and moiles to get a bit of that poisty, so as they shouldn't faul in these yere fits'.

A part of the gibbet post survived until the mid-1880s. When the original finally collapsed – in part because visitors, and also enterprising locals selling fragments to gullible visitors or at markets and fairs, had shaved away so much of its substance – the remains were taken to the local inn and it was replaced by a facsimile, the first of several, topped by an iron cockerel with the date 1734 inscribed into it. So far as is known, the facsimile was not believed to have curative virtues, and the trade in charms came to an end at about this time.

Though gibbets and the bodies on them were at the centre of nebulous constellations of popular cures, one of the most popular, and widely recorded, was in the treatment of goitre. Thus one traditional Sussex remedy for goitre or for a wen on the throat was the touch of a dead man's hand.

Mary Latham described how her childhood walks on Beeding Hill in the 1840s were spoilt by her terror at an ancient gibbet which stood there, and by the gruesome tales concerning it which her nurse insisted on recounting. One of these was about a woman who was cured of a wen on her neck by the touch of a dead murderer's hand: 'she was taken under the gallows in a cart and was held up in order that she might touch the dead hand, and she passed it three times over the wen, and then returned homewards.'

The nurse was not romancing. Here is a description of just such a scene at a public execution at Horsham, from a *Brighton Herald* of 1835:

'After the execution a circumstance occurred which excited much surprise that it should have been allowed to occur. This was the ancient and superstitious custom of passing the hand of the dead man while yet warm over the necks of two young females, by whose family this is considered as a remedy for diseases of the glands with which they are afflicted.'

For another curious cure for goitre, see **Viper**.

With the cessation of public hangings this gruesome procedure became impossible, and the original operation whereby the touch of a man hanged by the neck was used to cure conditions characterized by a swelling of the neck – the connection presumably being the squeezing and contracting of the throat inflicted on the hanged man and squeezing the life out of a swelling on the neck – was extended to include human corpses of every kind. The cure could also be effected by a 'hand of glory' or 'dead man's hand' carved out of a mandrake or false mandrake.

Note that gibbets were by no means rare in bygone Sussex. Convicted smugglers were gibbeted on the sea shore, and it was no uncommon sight on hill or cross roads or parish boundary to see the bodies of convicts hanging in chains in a gibbet cage or from the gallows until they decayed and fell down, or were devoured by ravens and kites.


# GLOW-WORM WINE

In 16th and 17th century Sussex glow-worms distilled or macerated in wine were a popular cure for both drunkenness and lust. An example of this comes from one of the no longer extant works of Leonard Mascall of Plumpton Place, Plumpton, East Sussex, as quoted in 1627 by John Goodyer, the Hampshire and West Sussex botanist:

'Glow-worms being drunk in wine make the use of lust not only irksome but loathsome. It was widely wisht therefore that the unclean sort of lechers were with frequent taking of these in Potion distill'd, who spare neither wife, widow, or maid, but defile themselves with lust not fit to be mentioned'.

## GREEN OYNTMENT

Timothy Butt of Tillington's *Book of Remedies* (1757) includes this curious 'receipt':

'How to Make Green Oyntment. One ounce of roseham. Half an ounce of beeswax, two ounces of turcomtine. Half an ounce of berdegrees. Beat it to a powder. Keep them sturd till they are all melted, then add to them 3 quarters of a pound of fresh grees. Keep it sturd till it is almost cold. For a green wound anoint it first with oil of turcomtine then apply the ointment.'

## HEDGEHOGS

Preparations made from badgers and hedgehogs were used throughout Sussex as cures for thinning or receding hair (presumably an example of sympathetic magic, using the hairy hedgehog, badger – or in Central Europe, bear! – to stimulate hair growth). An ointment made from the hindquarters of hedgehogs cooked and mixed with the fleed (inner fat) of pigs is the most frequently recorded treatment for baldness, mentioned in sources as far removed in time as the Revd Turner in 1685 and the Revd D.A. Gordon's *Selborne Notes* column in the 1890s.

And here is a recipe, originally from Turner, jotted down in the *Account and Memorandum Books* of the Stapley family of Hickstead Place, Twineham, in the 1730s:

'To cure the stone, though of long-standing, take a hedgehog and kill him, and flaw him, and wash the skin very clean, and then spread it out with something that will keep it at its full length. So stretched, dry it in the oven until the prickles will come off, which take and beat to a powder, and take the same powder in whatever liquor you drink.'

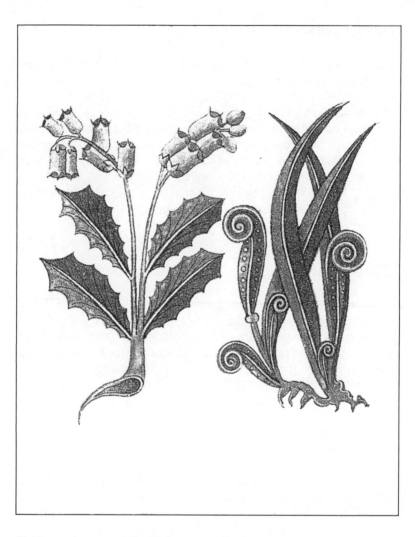

*Henbane, from an early 16th century English manuscript.*

# HENBANE
(Sussex dialect names Devil's Eye, Stinking Roger)

Henbane, *Hyoscyamus niger*, is a solenaceous plant found growing in shady places, particularly in overgrown quarries and around rubble and ruins everywhere in Sussex. It is related to mandrake and deadly nightshade, a plant rare in rural medicine because of its unpredictable and dangerous nature, though sometimes used in treating rabies (scc **Dog**).

Henbane contains in all its parts hallucinogenic, mind-altering, sleep, coma and death-inducing alkaloids such as hyoscine. Although an outright poisoning plant – henbane was the poison of Dr Crippen – it nonetheless had, in smaller doses, many applications in early and in country medicine as a source of pain-killing sleep-inducing drugs. Sussex people chewed on the roots to relieve toothache – this at a time when having teeth pulled was a terrifying ordeal – and bellyache; the bruised leaves were applied as bandages to soothe inflamed wounds (it was not strictly a woundwort, because not used to clean or close wounds, only to relieve pain). Together with opium and wine it was often an ingredient of the addictive, hallucinogenic pain-killing beverage laudanum, made in many households or available from apothecaries.

Finally here is an extraordinary late 17th century Sussex recipe: 'Children's Necklace for the Teeth' for teething pains which must have given harrassed mums many hours of untroubled leisure, containing henbane, one of our most potent analgesic, sleep, coma and death inducing plants, liberally soaked in alcohol:

'Take roots of henbane, of orpin and vervain and scrape them clean with a sharp knife, cut them in long beads and string them green, first henbane, then orpin, then vervain, till it is the bigness of the child's neck. Then take as much red wine as you think the necklace will take up and put thereto a dram of red coral, and as much single penny root finely powdered. Soak the beads in this for 28 hours and when red and dry, let the child wear and chew them.'

# HERRING, RED

On 3rd May 1671 the Revd John Allin, puritan vicar of Rye and dabbler in alchemy and astrology, wrote from London to his friend and fellow astrologer Mr Samuel Jeake of Rye:

'I hope yor son have long since lost his ague; if not, or any one else be much afflicted, this plaine and easy medicine have beene often tryed: for a man, or a woman; take 2 *red herrings* [ie cured or smoked]; for a child, but one red herring; take ye bones out well; yen sow it or them up in a thin cloth, with ye heads uppmost, and ye fleshy pte toward ye body; bind it or them upon ye reines [kidneys], and applye playsters and burgundy pitch to ye writs; this keepe on till well; or els renew as occasion serve.

'For yor sons hearing, if it yet be defective, take a leaf of coltsfoote and bruise it betweene yor fingers, and withall Juicye, make a kind of tent of it and putt it into ye eare troubled, and stop it after with wooll; and renew it as occasion serve.'

See also **Ague**.


# ILL WIND

It has frequently been remarked upon that the great majority of 16th and early 17th country houses and mansions in Sussex face resolutely north-east. This seems surprising, as those who built them generally had complete freedom when it came to choosing the desired aspect – which for us would be south or south-west for sunshine and balmy evenings. The probable reason why our ancestors opted for this aspect was explained by Robert Willis Blencowe in the 1920s. He writes about one old Elizabethan house – standing near the footpath which runs from a stone bridge near Paxhill to Horsted Keynes – which defies this rule:

84

'It stands upon an eminence, commanding a fine view, boldly fronting the west. Such it is well known, is not generally the case with our Sussex houses of that age; most of them lie immediately under the Downs, and look to the north and east. Shelter was, of course, in some degree, their object; but there was a prevalent notion in those days, and afterwards, that the south wind brought sickness on its soft wings and that the north and east winds were the harbingers of health...'

Thomas Tusser of East Hoathly, East Sussex, in his *Five Hundred Pointes of Good Husbandrie*, says:

'The south, as unkind, draweth sickness too near;
The north, as a friend, maketh all again clear.'

## INSECTS

A variety of insects were used in Sussex rural medicine; notably those containing or exuding a bitter, corrosive or irritant substance – ants, bees, bombardier and blister beetles. The underlying 'counter-irritant' principle was to produce stimulation or even blistering on the surface of the skin and thus, by stimulating blood flow, to remove toxins from, and relieve the congestion of, underlying tissues, thereby relieving conditions such as arthritis or rheumatism. The principle is valid in at least some of its applications, and is still applied in modern medicine.

Persistent skin conditions such as lupus and deeper-seated articulo-muscular conditions like arthritis and rheumatism were often treated by the external application of ants – held against the skin or enclosed in a frame tied to the skin – or the application of formic acid prepared by crushing etherized ants in a pestle and mortar. A writer in the *Sussex Daily News* in 1881, for example, described how, following a tradition deeply implanted among his neighbours in the Crowborough district, he applied jars of live wood ants – ferocious biters

– to his swollen arthritic joints, with effects which he deemed eminently satisfactory.

Such practices seem to have been discovered and rediscovered many times in primitive and folk medicine. For example, the Bolivian Indians championing of their ant stings in the treatment of arthritic and rheumatic conditions led a group of Canadian scientists to collect a million Bolivian ants for medical experimentation. Their work confirmed that the application of frames containing angry ants produced excellent results with some, but not all, forms of arthritis and rheumatism.

Bee venom, too, had an important place in Sussex rural medicine. Only recently the *Mid Sussex Times* related how a gardener living in Hailsham became so desperate for a means of relieving his rheumatism that he resorted to the painful but effective traditional remedy of applying enraged bees to his sore and swollen joints, apparently effecting a complete cure (I'd be wary of trying this one, because of the risk of potentially fatal allergic reactions to bee venom).

According to Leonard Mascall, the Plumpton Place agriculturist, writing in the 16th century, bee stings were also used as a cure for gout.

The blistering agent cantharidin obtained by crushing blister beetles of the *Meloidae* in a pestle and mortar was similarly used in the treatment of arthritis and rheumatism, and also, like the corrosive sap of many plants, for eating away warts (see **Warts**). It could be prepared at home or obtained from the apothecary – sometimes in the form of the notorious 'Spanish Fly', from the Spanish blister beetle *Lytta vesicatoria*, occasionally used as a potentially lethal aphrodisiac.


## INVENTORIES
### A Midhurst Surgeon and Petworth Tradesmen

Not one of the great Sussex diarists or correspondents of the 17th and 18th centuries was an apothecary or surgeon, so there is no one of that period to speak to us directly across the years, nobody to tell us what it was like to be a surgeon in Midhurst in 1740 or an apothecary in Cuckfield in 1720. For the most part they are shadow figures glimpsed only when diarists mention their visits to treat members of the family; through the bills they sent in for treatment of private individuals (cf the many household account books quoted elsewhere) or under the Poor Law. We also view them via their trade cards and advertisements; and when they are mentioned in contemporary documents as having taken on some function in the community, such as that of churchwarden. Finally in a glass darkly, via the inventories of their possessions which were compiled late in their lives or on their deaths. With the help of a little imagination, even these dry-as-dust inventories bring them to life and provide us with insights into what it was like to be a surgeon, barber-surgeon, physician, or apothecary in a small Sussex town in the 17th and 18th centuries.

In 1631, William White, surgeon in Midhurst, had goods valued at £180.17s.10d (I'll be setting down figures later which put this sum into context). A selection from a long and detailed inventory – published in full and discussed in F.W. Steer's *Medical History*, 1958 – includes: 'a pr of gould weights, 2 pr of scissors, a head brush, a pr of curling irons, and a hone: 7s; 1 Incision knife, 1 silver spatter, 1 sticking quill, a probe, a bodkin, a ladle, a steamer and a squirte, all silver: 20s; other tools of surgery with the box: 5s; 5 lancets, cirrenges and other tools: 16s. In the stilling loft: 3 stills, 1 flagon, 4 doz glasses, bottles, urinals and other glasses: 45s. His distilled waters, pothecary drugs and other like things: £3.6s.4d.'

He had two little hogs and a nag: £5. The lease of his house was of 'no value'. His library of books was valued at £10; he may well have had about 100 volumes. His wearing apparel and money in his purse was valued at £20. In the house he had two maps: 5s; a bastard musket, a halberd, a target and headpiece: 18s; his silver, which included a wine bowl, was valued at £15. The amounts of wine and measures in his inventory suggest that he sold wine and possibly tobacco, of which he had 16s worth. The wine stock was half a hogshead of sack and an almost full ditto: £12; three quarters of a hogshead of claret, a hogshead of white wine: £8; white wine: 50s; four pottle (half gallon) pots, six quarter pots, seven pint pots, one half pint pot, one pewter funnel, one little measure and a percer [piercer]: £2.18s.8d; ten wicker bottles, one glass bottle, two wine glasses: 7s; six empty wine vessels, two stands: 25s. He lived in comfort in a 13-roomed house, including the shop, having a wine and beer cellar. His desperate (bad) debts amounted to £10. No savings are mentioned.

From his total wealth, the house he lived in, and the variety and quality of his possessions and interests, it is clear that William White belonged to the wealthiest 5% of the Midhurst population. Like many surgeons he was a tradesman-cum-professional of some wealth and status – probably entitled to the appellation 'Mister' – and also of learning, perhaps with interests in subjects such as astrology and alchemy which today we would regard as esoteric. But though many surgeons were clearly men of substance and high status, not all surgeons, and not all medics, were as wealthy or, it would seem, as learned as William White.

The Petworth tradesmen's inventories compiled by J.H. Benson show that at any one time between 1600 and c1780 there were either one or two surgeons/barber-surgeons/physicians/or apothecaries practising in the town of Petworth. None was notably rich, only one is referred to as Mr, most have wealth and possessions which place them near the average for tradesmen – neither notably wealthy (in terms of contemporary money, that might mean inventory values of £150+ in 1620, £200+ in 1740), nor close to indigence.

J. Morris (Mr), Apothecary, 1721: total inventory £172 (for comparison with the White inventory, there had been some inflation during the previous century, so this is equivalent to perhaps £140 in the money of 1631); household goods £45, trade stock and tools £45, cash £5, money at interest, on bond or mortage £72, was owed debts of £5. The only tradesman of the time described as 'Mr'. He seems to have lived at the Dyehouse near the Market Place from 1680. His trade goods include seven dozen bottles, and he had two stills.

From the household accounts of the Dukes of Somerset at Petworth House, we know that in the late 17th and early 18th centuries he was called in to treat the family for a variety of ailments on a number of occasions (average bill, c £3), but when Lord Hertford, who died young, was seriously ill he was passed over in favour of a celebrated surgeon from London, who charged £32.

J. Haslen, Barber-Surgeon, 1667: Total inventory £112. Household goods £50, trade stock £21, cash £10, was owed £24. He was the Parish Registrar in 1653. The house had an apothecary's shop and a trimming shop, the former with £20 of drugs and medicines; the latter had two stills and a furnace. He had two rapiers, 12 red leather chairs, a marble stone for smoothing clothes, some books and a painted calico cloth, a well-furnished kitchen, some hogs, a nag, and hay valued at £3.

G. Haslen, Barber-Surgeon, 1682: Total inventory £39. Household goods £23, trade goods £4, cash £5. Possibly lived in the same house as J. Haslen, which was differently described or partly empty. In his shop were a case of instruments, books and medicines £4. Other goods include a birding piece, a 'coutch', a 'seeing glass', and a still.

H. Allen, Physician, 1614: Total inventory £42. Household goods £27, trade stock £2, cash £3, farm stock and coops £10. He is described as a 'Practicioner in Phisicke and Chirurgeria'. His trade stock included: 'Divers glasses of waters and pothecarys stuff 30s.2d, turner's tools, certain vials and glasses 10s'. He had a gelding and a little mare, a load of hay, saddles etc £10.7s.2d. He lived in fair comfort, having six beds, three pestles and mortars, one old still, two old books (3s), linen including damask table cloths worth £5.14s, one little silver bowl, eight silver spoons, a pewter aquavite bottle, a musket and a clock.

To put these inventory values into perspective, some 70

trades were represented in Petworth from cardboard makers to collar makers, chandlers and upholsterers. Several tradesmen were referred to as 'Mr', and several gentlemen were in trade. Inventory values were as follows: blacksmiths £40; 163; 55; 23; 257; 11; 44; 16; 151; 41; bricklayers £6; 46; 49; 21; 100; brickmaker £33; butchers £50; 23; 134; 36; 1,213; 683; 157; 98; carpenters £33; 35; 12; 47; 94; chapmen £215; 253; clerk £78; clothier £23; clothmaker £109; collier £55; cooper £422; cook £159; cordwainers £121; 39; 514; 65; curate £167; cutler £634; distiller £190; farriers £158; 29; flax dresser £207; fuller £44; gardeners £19; 50; glaziers £107; 70; glazier-plumber £61; glovers £77; 1; 539; 225; 1,477; haberdasher £618; host £3; innholders £271; 541; 116; 62; 29; 58; 131; 59; joiners £9; 54; keeper £295 [the head-keeper on the Petworth Estate, a lucrative and effectively hereditary post]; knacker £399; labourers £45; 27; locksmith £27; maltester £303; 484; 369; 26; 296; 202; 163; 139; masons £2; 35; 496; 6; mercers £570; 739; 1,737; 808; 259; millers £135; 49; 63; molecatcher £59; musicians £18; 49; saddlers £57; 31; sawyers £34; 69; 53; servants £2; 35; schoolmaster £165; shearmen £3; 4; 25; shoemakers £13; 40; 60; 96; 25; 180; staymakers £44; 28; tailors £38; 60; 32; 136; tanners £205; 119; 230; 252; tobacconists £57; 538; turners £69; 116; victuallers £40; 33; 18; vintner £78; weaver £30; wheelwrights £63; 1,038. Sundry 'Gentlemen' – almost by definition people who didn't have to stoop to 'trade', though some did – had inventories of £275; 129; 129; 284; 120; 0; 48; 935; 222; 100; 10; 634; 515.

# KING'S EVIL

Incidental entries on the flyleaves of early parish registers often repay investigation, for frequently they throw light on obsolete customs once prevalent. Among the most interesting are the incidental notes mentioning or listing the issue of Certificates for the Royal Touch for the cure of the King's Evil: certificates signed by the parish authorities, usually the minister and/or his churchwardens, confirming that a particular parishioner was indeed suffering from scrofula, the King's Evil, and hence might be entitled to take a day or more off from his labour to travel to London or some point on a royal 'Progress' through the country to have admittance to the king and receive the Royal Touch for the cure of that ailment.

The custom of touching by the sovereign for the cure of the scrofula, *Morbius Regius* or King's Evil, is traceable at least as far back as Edward the Confessor. There is evidence throughout the Middle Ages that English kings touched for this disease. Archbishop Bradwardine (the famous 'Doctor Profundus') who like his grandfather and father was a native of Chichester, in his celebrated work *De Causa Dei* alludes to documents speaking of past cures by the Royal Touch and of touches wrought in his own time.

Andrew Borde of Pevensey, in his *Breviary of Health* written during the reign of Henry VIII advises: 'for this matter let every man make Frendes of the Kynges Majestie, for it doth perteyne to a Kynge to helpe this Infirmitie by the Grace of God, the which is given to a Kynge anoynted'.

The eldest daughter of Henry VIII was our first queen regnant, and if it was questioned – as it seems to have been – whether the hands of a lady might be as efficacious as those of the many kings her forefathers, Mary had no scruples on that account, and did not long keep the practice in abeyance. In a letter found among the archives of Venice, the ceremony used by her is described by an eye witness. On Holy Thursday 1556 the feet washing by the Queen took place, when Bishop Day, of Chichester, the Grand Almoner, distributed alms to upwards of 3,000 people.

The next day 'she went to bless the scrofulous; but she chose to perform this act privately in a gallery where there was not above twenty persons . . . She caused one of the infirm women to be brought to her, when she knelt and pressed with her hands on the spot where the sore was. This she did to a man and three women. She then made the sick people come to her again, and taking a gold coin, viz an angel, she touched the place where the evil showed itself,

91

signed it with this coin, and passed a ribbon through the hole which had been pierced in it, placing one of them round the neck of each of the patients and making them promise never to part with that coin, save in case of extreme need.'

How long these were sometimes retained may be seen in an example of a 'touch piece' which passed through the hands of Elizabeth I and then passed from generation to generation in the family of Charles Austen Jacques of Chichester, who presented it to the Sussex Archaeological Society in the 19th century.

After the execution of Charles I, his blood-stained shirt and the sheet which covered his remains were long preserved in Ashburnham Church, East Sussex, and to these the Sussex peasantry repaired during many generations to obtain their touch for the King's Evil or other ills; the relics eventually being removed from the church to the house of the Ashburnham family, presumably because the popularity of the custom had become embarrassing.

As might be expected, after the Restoration, Charles II soon began to touch for the Evil, and was as readily resorted to by zealous royalists. He and the second James seem to have touched more than all their predecessors added together, and surviving sources referring to the issue of Certificates for the Royal Touch by Sussex parishes are mainly from the period 1660-1687.

In three Sussex registers, at least, those of Horsted Keynes, Wadhurst and Petworth, are preserved certificates or lists of certificates from this period, without which no applicant would have been admitted to Whitehall, and 'all ministers and churchwardens were required to be very careful to examine into the truth before they gave such'.

In 1746, while on a visit to the Revd Bush, vicar of Wadhurst, Dr Ducarel copied the following certificate from the register of the parish (*Nichol's Literary Anecdotes* 2,502):

'We the minister and churchwardens of the parish of Wadhurst, in the county of Sussex, do hereby certify that Mr Nicholas Barham, of this parish, aged about 24 yrs, is afflicted (as we are credibly informed) with the disease commonly called the King's Evil; and (to the best of our knowledge) hath not hitherto been touched by his Majestie for the said disease. In testimony whereof we have hereunto set our hands and seals this 23rd day of March 1684. John Smith, Vicar; Robert Longley, Thomas Yonge, Churchwardens.'

On the flyleaf at the end of the earliest register for Petworth occurs a list of 38 'Certificates for his Majesty's Sacred Touch ordered to bee Registered in 1683' and then '1685-8'.

The number of persons thus touched by Charles II during the last ten years of his reign was no fewer than 90,798 which would be almost incredible, were it not attested by a record kept by the Keeper of the Closet. Evelyn, a spectator, observed that the king stroked 'their faces or cheeks with both his hands at once', and in his diary (28 March 1684) Evelyn mentions a dreadful accident: that 'there was so great a concourse of people with their children to be touched for the evil, that 6 or 7 were crushed to death by pressing at the chirurgen's door for tickets'.

Thereafter William III refused to touch (although Whiston says that he once did so, and that the patient was saved). Queen Anne frequently touched; Barrington mentions questioning an old man in Mayfield who, when a child, was touched by her. He asked him whether he was really cured, upon which the old man answered with a significant smile, that 'he believed himself to have never had a complaint that deserved to be considered as the Evil, but that his parents were poor, and had no objection to the bit of gold'.

The Duke of Monmouth and the Old Pretender both touched, but the sovereigns of the House of Brunswick from George I onwards seldom or never did so and the custom fell into disuse; though scrofulaics repaired to the relics of Charles I at Ashburnham throughout the 18th century.

Travelling to London to be touched by the king was – for reasons not difficult to divine – the most sought after recourse for scrofula sufferers, but when this was not possible, and after the cessation of the tradition, country people turned to herbal treatments which usually involved

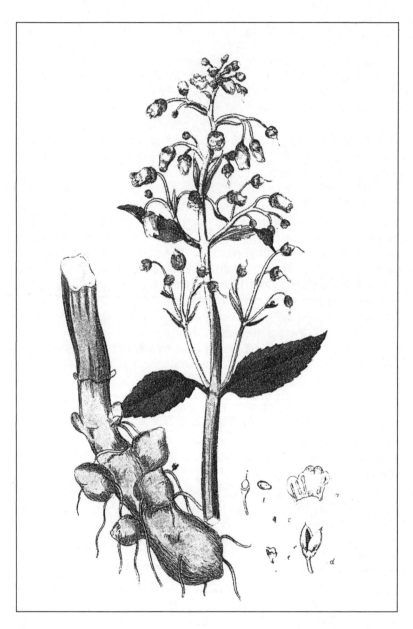

*Figwort, from* Flora Medica, *1829*

the plants known as figworts, namely the lesser figwort or lesser celandine, *Ranunculus ficaria*, and the unrelated greater figwort *Scrophularia nodosa*.

Sussex dialect names for lesser celandine – angel, brighteye, butter-and-cheese, butterchops, cheesecups, cream and butter, dillicup, figwort, fogwort, foxwort, golden cups, goldyknob, kingcup, king's evil, pilewort, powerweed, rose noble, starlight – clearly fall into two main groups, the obvious names inspired by the beautiful butter-yellow flowers; and a second family harking back, more obscurely, to the plant's uses in the herbal era.

In 1548, William Turner made the first mention of lesser celandine or figwort as a British plant: 'Figwort groweth under the shaddowes of ashe trees'. It was figwort or pilewort – whence also fogwort, foxwort, powerweed – because the nodular root tubers were, according to the Doctrine of Signatures, a signature indicating its efficacy as a cure for 'the fig' (Latin *ficus*, whence *ficaria*), ie for piles:

> 'the later age use the rootes and grains for the fig or piles; which being often bathed with the juice mixed with wine, or with the sick man's urine, are drawne together and dried up and the paine quite taken away' (Gerard, 1597)

For the same reason, it also cured 'kernels by the ears and throat, called the King's Evil', whence the local names angel, king's evil, kingcup, and rose noble; angels and rose nobles being the coins bearing the king's effigy bestowed by the king at a touching or sometimes used to cure the Evil in lieu of the king's own touch.

> 'Let the good people make much of it for these uses,' wrote Culpeper, 'with this I cured my own Daughter of a King's Evil, broke the Sore, drew out a quarter of a pound of Corruption, cured it without any scar at all, and all in one week's time'

A second plant known in Sussex as figwort, pilewort, king's evil and rose noble was the greater pilewort or greater figwort. Another plant for the fig or piles, another signature plant, the knobs or protuberances on the roots signifying that it had been placed on Earth as a cure for both piles and the kernels or tubercular glands of the King's Evil, whence two further local names apparently exclusive to it: kernelwort and throatwort.

Piles, the King's Evil, ulcers, sores, cancers, and even sore and red faces were all treated with this rather ugly, brown-flowered and smelly herb, which was widely used in Sussex rural medicine until the early 19th century. The Revd Turner writing in the late 17th century gives the recipe for a 'plaister' for the Evil made of greater figwort and hound's-tongue leaves and the flowers of foxglove and white dead-nettle.

Around Crowborough and Tunbridge Wells, greater figwort was known, until well into the present century, as crowdy kit, or fiddlewort. A crowdy was an olden-time fiddle; children made a squeaky fiddler's noise by scraping one dry stem of figwort across another.

# LEECH-CATCHER, THE

The leech-catcher, like the herb woman, the mandrake man, the toad-eater, and the viper-catcher, was a familiar figure in the Sussex of yesteryear.

From the Middle Ages through to the late 19th century, incalculable numbers of leeches were used by doctors, surgeons, and hospitals for 'bleeding' patients; an operation which might also be carried out using surgical instruments.

The practice of bleeding, almost universal among the wealthier and middle classes and dependents such as live-in employees as well as in hospitals and almshouses, seems to have been less popular among poorer sections of the population – though blacksmiths, farriers, cunning folk and others deemed to have mechanical or medical skills could earn a useful supplementary income by bleeding the wealthier at prices which undercut apothecaries, barber-surgeons, and surgeons. Their advantage was not only in price but (in outlying rural areas at least), in being local and thus better placed than licensed medics, most of whom were based in towns, to carry out a commonplace operation which was the standard response to many ailments and psychological states. It was also in early times at least, part of the hygiene of everyday life.

On 24th May 1735, for example, Richard Stapley of Hickstead Place, Twineham, noted in the family's Account and Memorandum Books: 'James Matthew [the local farrier] did let me blood in my left foot, and it was the fourth time that I had been so blooded. And he let my wife blood in the right arm the next day.'

In the 17th century John, First Lord Ashburnham, wrote to his agent in London asking him to engage a valet 'who must be between 30 and 40 years of age and skilled in letting blood and playing in the music'.

And the Household Account Books of the Dacres of Herstmonceux Castle for 1643-9 list many small payments to local people for bleeding members of the family or household. For instance 'Paid Mr Walters for letting T.Christians blood 01s'.

As the Stapley entry hints, initially there were complex rules governing leeching. In the Middle Ages and until the 17th or early 18th centuries there were days of each month – determined from year to year by complex astrological calculations – when it was appropriate or imperative to let blood, and others when bloodletting was strongly disadvised (see **Cowfold, Churchwardens' Accounts**). This calender could be affected by one's birth day or birth sign, which may explain why Mr and Mrs Stapley were bled on different days. These Byzantine leeching calculations slowly passed from fashion during the 18th century, in parallel with the decline in astrology; to be replaced either by regular bleeding weekly or monthly as a means of keeping the body and its humours in equilibrium, or occasional leeching in response to particular ailments or states of health or mind (a feeling of heaviness; melancholy, excessive choler, etc).

It was also important to bleed from the right part of the body if the operation was to have the desired effect on the balance and spatial distribution of the four 'humours'. A 17th century doctor's bill found in the parish chest at Sedlescombe includes an item for bleeding a child under the tongue. The Stapley entry mentions bleeding Mrs Stapley from the right arm; and Richard Stapley from his left foot; bleeding from the feet being based on the notion that this drew the peccant humours downwards, and so was the best way of relieving disorders of the head and upper body.

Most leeches were collected in the field by professional or semi-professional leech-catchers who sold them to physicians, hospitals, blacksmiths/farriers or other local bleeders, or to an apothecary for resale. The most common method was to wade bare-legged into a pool or stream and allow the parasites to affix themselves.

Leech-catching was also a useful source of pocket money for boys and of supplementary income for agricultural labourers. Here is Thomas Parsons writing in 1934 about *Chichester 60-65 Years Ago*:

'The stream of the Lavant ran through the city behind some of the houses where the present Market Road now is, and formed an open ditch, beside which was a pathway leading to the fields. These were known as the Hunston Meadows. In the dry season this ditch was the receptacle for refuse, dead cats and dogs; and in the winter it became a rapid running stream passing under the road at Southgate into the fields on the south-western end of the city, known as the Bishop's Fields. Following the line of the Roman wall, it eventually discharged into the sea at Appledram. We could collect from the arches, through which it ran, a large number of leeches, and as bleeding was at that time very popular with the medical profession and no chemist's shop was complete which did not contain a bowl of these creatures, the collecting of them was a source of income to the boys who could sell them to the chemists for a few pence.'

*Hirudo medicinalis'* rarity as a wildling in the British Isles today renders these methods no longer practicable, although over-collecting is probably only one factor in its decline and disappearance. Others would seem to be the loss of its pond and stream habitat, as well as the increasing scarcity of creatures such as common frogs which constitute one of the parasite's favoured hosts when it cannot find mammals.

Nowadays the most tangible memory we have left of what was once a major industry lies in the handsome decorated porcelain, often Delftware, jars in which leeches were kept for sale in oldentime apothecaries' shops.

Modern research has shown that moderate leeching can be beneficial in certain conditions where the blood is 'too thick' – but the evidence from 14th-18th century sources suggests that the benefits, where these existed, were often outweighed by the dangers of being bled to death by over-enthusiastic doctors ready to prescribe bleeding as the cure for just about any and every ailment.


# LIVESTOCK REMEDIES

Cattle, sheep, pigs, horses and chickens were of an importance that cannot be overstated in the rural economy of yesteryear. For an agricultural labourer or smallholder the possession of a small plot for growing vegetables and of a cow, a couple of pigs or a few hens, could represent the difference between abject poverty – the inescapable lot of any family that was solely dependent on a farm labourer's wage – and tolerable survival. Already true in Elizabethan times it became increasingly so as rural wages fell steeply in real terms, and tracts of once common land around villages were enclosed, denying access to wild salads, vegetables, fruit and game, and also tightening the noose on smallholding by reducing communal pannage (the right to pasture pigs in a forest) and grazing for sheep and cattle. The loss of such family livestock to disease could be, almost literally, a mortal blow. More solidly rooted husbandmen or yeomen farmers were often gravely inconvenienced by the loss of a valuable animal, or brought close to ruin if their livestock was afflicted

The Government of

# CATTEL.

*Divided into three Books.*

The firſt, Treating of Oxen, Kine, and Calves: and how to uſe Bulls, and other Cattel, to the yoke or fell.

The ſecond, Diſcourſing of the Government of Horſes; with approved Medicines againſt moſt Diſeaſes.

The third, Diſcourſing of the Order of Sheep, Goats, Hogs, and Dogs; with true Remedies to help the Infirmities that befall any of them.

Alſo, Perfect inſtructions for taking of Moals; and likewiſe for the monthly Husbanding of Grounds: and hath been already approved, and by long experience entertained a-mongſt all ſorts; eſpecially Husbandmen, who have made uſe thereof, to their great profit and contentment.

Gathered by LEONARD MASCAL.
*Chief farrier to King* J A M E S,

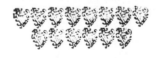

*Title page from Mascal's* The Government of Cattel, 1662. *(Sussex Archaeological Society Library)*

100

by disease. So it comes as no surprise that cunning women or, more commonly, cunning men with skills in treating animals were in great demand, the most successful earning themselves a reputation as 'cow doctors', 'horse doctors', and so on. Farmers too were assiduous collectors of remedies or charms for treating or protecting stock; jotting them down in the margins of account and husbandry books.

Here are a few examples of recipes and charms noted in the account books of Timothy Butt, a barely literate small farmer at Tillington, between 1765 and 1800:

'For a horse that hath the Fashons – Take one ounce of Anniseeds one ounce of Turmerick one ounce of Birthwort all powders. Of Vinill Lungwort Arbegrass Wormwood Read Sage. Shreed them all small and take of each one handfull and lay a steep in 3 Quarts of Spring Water let then lye 24 hours all those will make 3 Drenches and ye second many Bleed.'

'For a bulluck that is Sprung – say these Words. Our Blesed Saviour for his Sons sake Pray Down the Blader, Blow that he may break. In the name of the Father and of the Son and of the Blessed Trinitey Saved may this Black Bulluck be – or let the Collet [colour] be what it will Name it. Then say the Lords Prayer and so say it 3 times.'

'For a Bulluck that is Stung with an Adder – take Salt and fresh Grees and anoynt the Beast for the heart of them say these Words – Simon Joan Heart why couldn't thou thy Sarvant thou stungest thou my man. I wish it were thy man take Salt and Smare and lay to the Speer. In the Name of the Father and of the Son and of the Holy Ghost Amen.'

This last is a very fine piece of gibberish from which no amount of textual gloss, interpretation or deconstruction seems likely to extract any sense.

'For a bite of a Mad Dogge' . . . see **Dogs**
'For a Strain or a Bruse . . .' see **Swallow Water**.
'Eye Water – One Quartern of White Port half a Quarter of an ounce Collimeney Stone powdered put into the

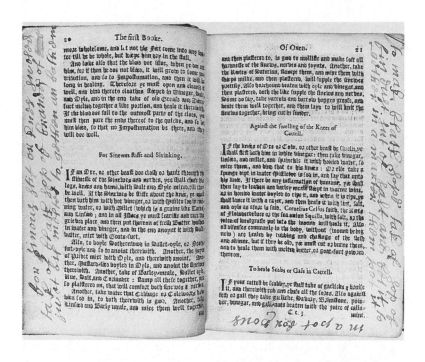

*Pages from* The Government of Cattel *showing a Sussex yeoman farmer's annotations. (Sussex Archaeological Society Library)*

Bottle of Wite wine then for a Bulluck's Eye blow some of the Powder in, but if it be a Christons Eye then wash it with the Water.'

And here are examples of remedies jotted into a 4th edition of *The Government of Cattel*, by Leonard Mascal of Plumpton, East Sussex, which was published in 1662 and passed through the hands of many generations of Sussex yeomen farmers and country gentlemen (several of whom inscribed their names in the book) before being obtained for the library of the Sussex Archaeological Society in 1895. The annotations, in several different hands, are undated and difficult to decipher but are probably from the period 1662-1760.

On the front flyleaf is 'A Drink for the Yallows in A Bollock – take of Sullandine, of Fetherfew, of yarb, Agrase, of Shipard's Posh [pouch, or purse], of Peniriall, of Ishop [hyssop], of Bollock's Longwort, of Angellure. Take a pennard [pennyworth] of Anniseed, a pennard of Lickerstick [liquorice], a pennard of Carreway sed, a pennard of Coming [cumin] sed, some Persley sed, a pennard of Treakle. Boil it in Bear [beer] and give it blod warme.'

On the 2nd front flyleaf: 'A metsun [medicine] for the Yallows in a Sow. Take 1 penniwarth of Menerisk, 1 pennard of Safurant [saffron], 1 of lickersticks, 1 of Treckel, 1 of Anniseeds, 1 of Tunbrick [tumeric?], 1 hanful of Sullandine, 1 hanful of Goos dung. Buil it in bear and give it Luk warme.'

On the other side of leaf: 'To kil a . . ? Take of Bai salt, of Nettel sed, and stamp it, of Tar and Gun pouder and mex it al to gether.'

On the margin of a page: 'To the Reader. For the Reumatex in Man or Best. Take a hanful of Yar [yarrow?], an a hanful of fetherfoi [feverfew], and shredd smal, and boil them in fresh grece to an ointment, and bath the plas hot with it.'

On the margin of p12: 'To stop a Scouering in a Best. Take an ouns of Dragons blod, and a hanful of Yar and buil in milk and give it to the calf.'

Dragon's blood was a Sussex name for Herb Robert, *Geranium robertianum*; but in this context is more likely to be the apothecary's drug *Sanguis draconis* variously a bright red resin exudate from the fruit of the palm *Calamus draco*, or exudates from *Pterocarpus draco* or *Croton draco*.

On margin p13: 'For bluid passing. Take a hanful of holli-beries and bouil in milk and give it to the Best or Man or follers [Fullers] earth builed in milk.'

Margin p20: 'For Sinous [sinews] staf or Knes swolled. Take of black Sop, of Branee of swet Oil, melted together an bath em.'

Margin p21: 'To mak black Sope. Take of Sop, of fine dust Sut [soot] of Salt, and bet it to gether in a marter, then pot it in a pot for use.'

On margain p137: 'To swaig [assuage] a sweling in a Hors boddy. Sok a (?) of Branee, of swet Oil, of black Sop – buil it and bath the plas hot with it'.

On the two fly sheets at the end of the book: 'To make Besilican to hele soars in Man or Best. Take of Muten seuet [mutton suet] of black Peech [pitch] of Bees wax, of Rosam [rosin] of swet Iel [sweet oil] mext all to gether in a pot.'

In a different hand: 'Anguentum Diapomphalig to Dry a Sore'. In another hand 'angweritom Pomfuligust'. A third writes 'Unguentum Diapomphalig', then 'Pumpillian Ile of the Ile of Adder spear [probably adder's tongue fern] is Good for a cow erder [udder] sealed. And for the Rumatism Batesmans dropes'.

And lastly, the following names appear: 'James Summers his Book 1763. Mary Marchant her Bok 1767. Nicholas Marchant his book.'


## LUCKY STONES

In 16th-18th century Sussex sources there are several references to the use of perforated 'lucky stones' suspended from the dewlap to protect cattle from hags and pixies and the conditions they were believed to inflict (cf Mr H.S. Toms: *Sussex Notes and Queries* 1,232). Though the custom had apparently died out by the 19th century, in rural areas it remained commonplace to tie a piece of knotted twine through a hole in the ears or dewlap of cattle, though the reasons for doing so had been forgotten. For example this in *Sussex Notes and Queries* 2,147):

'Until quite recently, certainly within the last ten years, there was prevalent in the more pagan parts of the Forest Ridge in East Sussex the practice of piercing the dewlaps of young stock as a means of protecting the animals against being 'struck'. The disease thus warded off is known, I believe, to veterinary surgeons as symptomatic anthrax, which attacks thriving young animals so suddenly and so fatally as to suggest, no doubt, in earlier times the agency of a witch.

'The weanyer [newly weaned] animal when he was first turned out to graze had the dewlap perforated, and through the hole was run a piece of string, preferably tarred string, but a bootlace would do. The string was then tied in a knot and as far as I know remained in the dewlap until it perished and fell away. At any of the markets in those parts of the Weald indicated above a considerable proportion of the young stock offered for sale might be seen to have pierced dewlaps, or to be carrying the prophylactic twine, and it may well be that the custom still persists.

'Many of the ancient remedies and practices in use in the countryside have sound sense and much practical experience behind them, but none of those who applied the tarred string could give me any reason for doing so beyond the fact that it was the custom and a practice which he did not like to neglect. It seems possible that here is a survival of the use of the 'lucky stones' which used to be attached to the weanyer to prevent his being struck, and that the string which once was passed through the stone continued to be inserted into the dewlap long after faith in the stone had died and been forgotten.'

Whether or not the knotted twine was a direct descendent of the lucky stone, knots were in themselves widely held to be an effective defence against witches, hags, pixies, and the devil in all his manifestations. I suspect, too, that the twine through the dewlap could have been the survival of a sister custom. By ancient prescription the two native hellebores, the green *Helleborus viridis* and the stinking *H.foetidus* and also the widely cultivated Christmas rose *H.niger*, were used as remedies for cattle. When a cow wheezed or coughed, an issue was made through its dewlap with a needle and thread, and a length of the hellebore root was inserted and held in place by the thread to irritate or counter-irritate the flesh and keep it running, whence the hellebore's Sussex dialect name of oxheal.

# MANDRAKE

To understand the curious place of mandrakes, false mandrakes and mandrake men in the history of Sussex rural medicine, we must go back deep into the history of the mandrake legend.

The mandrake or mandragora *Mandragora officinalis* is native to the Mediterranean and Near and Middle East. Above ground, it appears a relatively innocent ordinary plant. The deep green leaves spread out in a flat rosette, interlaced with heavily-scented violet-tinged flowers. During late summer, the flowers ripen into deep golden berries with a sickly, troubling odour of musk.

Below ground, the mandrake is less innocent. Its forked double or triple black root is over a yard in length and, to an impressionable imagination at least, shaped like a man, a woman, a distorted simulacre, or a mannikin. The flesh of this dark man-like root is crammed with poisonous tropane alkaloids which have a soporific, pain-killing, dream, hallucination and sleep-inducing effect in small doses, but which bring on delirium, madness, coma and death in larger doses – mandrake was the poison of Lucrezia Borgia. All of which comes as no surprise, as the mandrake is a member of the *Solenaceae*, which includes such native poisoners as henbane and deadly nightshade.

The narcotic effects are there for a prosaic purpose: to protect food reserves in the root from the insects that dig galleries in carrots and potatoes. The unsuspecting insect that bites into a mandrake slides into a drugged sleep from which it never wakes.

Early Mediterranean peoples, unaware of this prosaic context, credited the man-shaped mandrake with mysterious powers. It was *the* plant of power in ancient medicine and magic.

Mandragora was first used as a surgical anaesthetic in Persia, three millenia ago. Before an operation or the removal of a tooth, a dried anodyne of mandragora and camphor was reconstituted in boiling water and a steaming sponge held at the patient's nostrils till he slumbered.

106

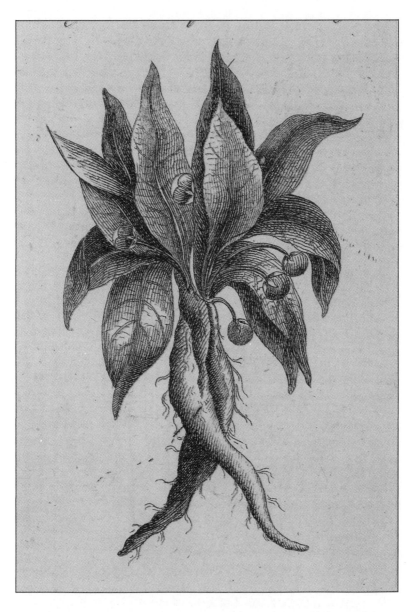

*An illustration of* Atropa Mandragora, *showing its bifurcated root.*
*(Mansell Collection)*

Mandrake was brought to and grown in Britain during Roman times. By the 8th century AD, Anglo-Saxon 'Leeches' were using mandragora as a painkiller and anaesthetic. The *Leech Books of Bald and Cild* tell us 'this wort is mickle and illustrious and it is beneficial'. ['Mickle' = great, magnificent; illustrious = luminescent; mandrakes were believed to glow like the moon at night.]

But though they used it in their medicine, the ancients were troubled by this root shaped like a man which had power over sleep, dreams, madness and death and grew amid plants of ill-repute such as ivy and yew. For the Greeks, it was the plant of Hecate, mistress of the Underworld: goddess of unquiet and oppressive dreams, nightmares, epilepsy, and madness. Greek legends tell of the quest for the mandragora which led to Hypnos, island of sinister dreams 'where nothing but tall poppies riot and mandragora sweet and sickly blooms, where silent butterflies float and no birds sing.'

Mandrake was also sacred to the Moon Goddess Selene because it was the plant of madness – and madness (lunacy), with reason, was linked with the Moon. With its musky smell, man or woman-like shape and power to induce visions and hallucinations it was the most powerful of all aphrodisiacs, as in the story of Leah in the Bible.

In medieval Europe, Hecate and Selene's plant – if it *was* a plant? – with its power to poison slowly and almost imperceptibly, to induce strange visions, and to send its victims mad, became of rights *the* witching plant, the plant of sorcery and evil. When torn from the ground it was said to emit screams which could send the listener mad. Shakespeare knew of this tradition, writing of

'Shrieks like Mandrake's torn out of the earth,
That living mortals, hearing them, run mad.'

*Romeo and Juliet*, Act IV Scene 3

and of its aphrodisiac and sleep-inducing powers:

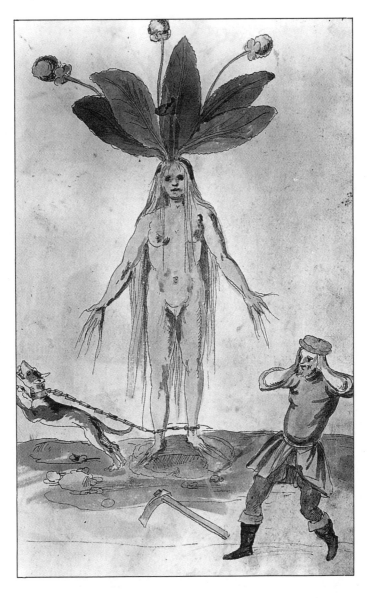

*A 16th century wash drawing of a dog unearthing a human-like mandrake while its master blocks his ears against the fabled unearthly shriek. (Mansell Collection)*

'Give me to drink mandragora, that I might sleep out this great gap of time.'

*Anthony and Cleopatra*, Act 1, Scene 5

Mandrakes were widely grown in English gardens during the medieval and Tudor periods. From the 15th century onwards mandrakes could be found hanging in the windows of Sussex apothecaries or draped over the shoulders of the mandrake men who peddled mandrakes from fair to fair, village to village. Some of those buying mandrakes were buying relief from pain or insomnia. Some, perhaps the majority, were seeking control of the mandrake's aphrodisiac or magical powers: dreams and visions, a reputedly infallible aphrodisiac, a slow poison with which they could kill a neighbour's cow or send a relative mad, or a means of casting spells of infallible power. Andrew Borde of Pevensey, writing in the early 16th century, mentions mandrake men who travelled from village to village with mandrakes dressed like dolls in fine clothes. At each stopping place they bathed their simulacres in milk, selling the resulting magical bath water to gullible people who believed they were buying control of dark satanic powers.

But mandrakes do not grow well in English conditions. Even in the mild, sunny Middle Ages up to the 15th century the native supply had always been limited; with the onset of the 'Little Ice Age' in the mid-16th century – which brought with it the great Frost Fairs on the Thames – the native supply dried to a trickle. Mandrakes were imported from Southern Europe but we know from the account books of importers that they were literally worth their weight in gold. So it is not surprising that mandrakes were widely counterfeited, particularly as there were two native look-alikes to hand in the black and white bryonies.

The black bryony *Tamus communis* is common in Sussex, though lost among other hedgerow plants for much of the year. It is a climber whose stem twines and winds its way around other hedgerow plants, turning in a clockwise direction as it follows the sun. Above ground it has no resemblance to a true mandrake, but it does have a large, dark, sometimes forked root which, while less man-like than that of true mandrake, can be carved into the shape of a man. The root is laced with bitter protective substances which possess medicinal virtues, but not the powers of true mandrake.

The unrelated white bryony *Bryonica dioica* or devil's turnip thrives on chalk, and is locally common in hedgerows on the Sussex Downs. Its tough, hairy stems climb by means of coiled tendrils, the plant supporting itself on hedgerow bushes as it makes its way upwards towards sunlight.

It was named with the black bryony because of its above-ground form and a large, often forked root – lighter in colour, whence the distinction between black and white – laced with bitter principles. Again, the roots possess none of the powers of real mandrake.

From Tudor times, black or white bryony roots cut into the shape of a man, with grains of millet inserted into the face as eyes, were passed off as 'mandrakes' fetching high prices. In his *Niewe Herball* (1562), Turner alludes to these 'pupettes' which are 'so trymmed of crafty thieves to mocke the poore people withall and to rob them of theyr wit and theyr money'.

According to Charles Johnson's *British Poisonous Plants* (1861), bryony mandrakes in human form, sown with grass to give them hair, were sold by Sussex apothecaries until into the 19th century; and naturalist Maurice Burton remembered seeing a black bryony mandrake in the window of an apothecary-cum-pharmacist during a visit to Ditchling just after the First World War.

From a very early date there is almost total confusion between real and mock mandrakes. When old sources mention mandrakes being sold by apothecaries or by travelling mandrake men, there is usually no way of knowing whether the mandrakes were real (given the scarcity of the supply probably only a small proportion, most of which probably went to wealthy people with esoteric interests) or black or white bryony pupettes. The earliest English herbalists record mandrake (and sometimes womandrake) as names for black and white bryony, and it is clear that black and white bryonies were known as 'mandrakes' from a very early time. Nor can we know how many of those who bought bryony 'mandrakes' were deceived into believing they were buying the mysterious powers of real mandrakes (quite a high proportion in early times, from the indignation of authors like Turner?), and how many were simply buying a local herb which had come to be called 'mandrake' for its much humbler virtues in human and horse medicine. One can, however, imagine that even bryony mandrakes which were bought knowingly as bryony roots must have carried some sort of aura not possessed by other herbs by virtue of the name and its associations lost in the mists of time.

Both the bryonies were said to be powerful aphrodisiacs, presumably because of their association with real mandrakes – one can't imagine such bitter purging plants possessing real aphrodisiac powers! Both were used as violent purges for worming children. Culpeper notes that they 'purge the belly with great violence' and 'burn the liver and therefore are not rashly to be taken'. He advises their use for curing palsies, cramps, stitches in the side, dropsy, kidney stones, bronchitis, internal bruising, fretting and running cankers, gangrene and tetters (skin complaints). They also, applied externally, were reputed to clear up black or blue spots, freckles, morphew, leprosy, scabs, splinters, and even broken bones, whitlows, warts, and sores. He repeatedly urged that bryony root needed 'an abler hand to correct them than most country people have'.

Bryony mandrakes were also much in demand for treating horses. Here, for example, is Mark Williamson, Warden of the Kingley Vale Nature Reserve, in his column in the *Chichester Observer*:

'I remember Fred Longman of Biderton, who once managed 700 acres of the chalk downs with horses, telling me that to put a horse in good condition, to make its coat bloom, the carters used to feed a small amount of mandrake grated up with the oats. Fred maintained that mandrake could be found here and there in the hedgerows in the farm at Lavant. Whether he meant the black or white

112

bryony I never did find out, but what is certain is that he meant one or other of the two plants, which for centuries have been known to herbalists as mock or false mandrakes. The medicine had to be administered sparingly, for the animal became extremely frisky, verging on wildness.'

Here we are plainly in the domain of straightforward rural medicine, far removed from real mandrakes and their strange powers.

The ambient rural confusion between real and mock mandrakes is well conveyed in the latest account I have come across of a Sussex mandrake man, in the *Sussex County Magazine* in 1929. The little old man is selling bryony mandrakes which he has collected himself in the Sussex hedgerows. They have not been carved into mandrake form and were prescribed, without any attempt at deception (or maybe just a teeny little bit), for the cure of minor ailments. But as would many of his customers, he is clearly confusing his bryony mandrakes with the real mandrakes of history and their mysterious powers, and is obviously aware of the legend concerning the way mandrakes shriek when torn from the soil:

' "This, sir," said the affable little old man in answer to my query concerning the queer root-like objects that, linked by a piece of stout twine, hung on each side of one of his broad shoulders, "this is a mandrake, the finest cure in all the world fer indigestion an' malaria, not a'mentionin' one or two other things which I won't guarantee, such as rheumatism, pains in the chest, 'ead-aches, and so on. I've been a'sellin of this 'ere stuff fer over 55 years now; an' I've got 'undreds of people all over the place who absurlootly swear by it. Try a bit yerself, sir." He fished in a tattered pocket and, producing a worn table knife, he cut a lump from one of the roots and held its moist white surface for me to examine.

"There ye are, sir. This 'ere root contains quin-ine and iron, and that's what makes it so good. All ye 'as to do is to scrape off its surface enough to cover a sixpence, an' put it in yer tea or whatevert else you might be a'drinkin'. Just that, sir, and it'll make a noo man of yer."

"Where do I get it?"

"Well, that's a secret, like, but I knows where to look for it. I tramps all over the place, sometimes fer days, diggin' under 'edges and in ditches, an' I 'as to search real 'ard, for the mandrake aint got no 'ead and don't show above ground. At times I 'as to dig nearly six feet down, and you should 'ear the row it kicks up when I pulls it out. Groans like anything it does.

"Sometimes I'm lucky enough to git a root as weighs over 60 pounds, but it always 'as to be the male root. The female aint no good at all. Funnily enough, though, if ye digs out the female root an' leaves the male, the male dies.

"'Ow old are they? Let's 'ave a look at this one' ere." He counted the rings upon it. "This one's about 120 year old, but most of 'em that I finds are over an 'undred.

"Mandrake's got a wunnerful 'istory, sir. It's the only 'erb as is mentioned in the Bible while Shakespeare talks about it several times in 'is plays. It was supposed to be used in magic and in makin' love potions in the old days, and people also thought as 'ow it caused madness an' even death. That's all bunkum, though. I wouldn't be allowed to traipse all over the country with it if it didn't do what I says it would, would I?

"Don't forget to try it sir. It'll do ye real good. Good-day sir, I'm just a'goin' over to the pub to get 'alf a pint." '


# MICE

It's difficult to understand why mice were a highly popular prescription for all sorts of ailments, except for the practical fact that they were easily obtainable and, it is said, quite palatable. They had many uses in Sussex rural medicine: fried or stewed with onions or roasted as a cure for consumption and whooping cough and also for diphtheria; baked to a cinder, powdered and mixed with jam, they could cure a child of bed wetting; dried and powdered they were good for diabetes.

Here is a typical recipe noted down in the Account and Memorandum Books of the Stapley family of Hickstead Place, Twineham, in 1734:

'To cure the hooping cough...Get 3 field mice, flaw them, draw them, and roast one of them, and let the party afflicted eat it; dry the other two in the oven until they crumble to a powder, and put a little of this powder in what the patient drinks at night and in the morning'.

That the little Stapleys of Twineham had derived benefit from this singular remedy can be confirmed by the fact that it is subscribed by *Approbatum Est* – tried and approved.

As recently as 1939, Dr P.H. Lulham wrote in the *Sussex County Magazine* that a few years previously, during an outbreak of diphtheria he had found out that some mothers were taking their children to a local wise woman. She would first tie a hazel twig round their throats, for which she charged a shilling, and then, if that failed, she would make them swallow a bit of stewed mouse while she recited an incantation, for which she charged half a crown. The doctor got the police to put a stop to her cures.

Mice were such a commonplace of folk medicine that there was a joke current in Sussex at one time about a doctor who was treating a child with high fever. He told the mother to put some ice in a bag on the child's forehead; next day she reported gratefully that the cure had worked: 'He's much better now, sir; the fever has gone down and the mice are dead'.

The woman – if the story was based on a real incident, which is quite probable – clearly believed in the transference of disease to suitable scapegoat plants or animals by contact. Such transfers were most likely to be successful if there was some obvious affinity between the plant or animal and the disease, as in the traditional practices of eating or wearing shivery, shiver-inducing spiders for the shivery ague, tying the shivery ague to shivering, trembling aspen trees, or using warty toads as suitably attractive scapegoats for the transfer of warts.

# MOULDS

Soon after the appearance of penicillin, medical historians began a search of the early literature to see if records of the use of this antibiotic could be found which predated Alexander Fleming's original 'official' discovery in 1928.

These studies soon showed that moulds similar to those from which we obtain penicillin had been widely used as curatives in folk medicines as far removed in time and place as Ancient Greece, Ancient China, and 16th-19th century Sussex.

A Greek king of the 16th century BC, for example, described how a peasant woman used mould scraped from mouldy cheese to treat his wounded soldiers; the Chinese, 3,000 years ago, used mouldy soya beans to treat infected cuts, wounds, and burns.

Long before Europeans arrived in Australia, aborigines were using moulds taken from the sheltered side of eucalyptus trees to treat wounds. Charles Kelleway, Director of the Eliza and Walter Hill Institute in Melbourne, remarks that a bushman once brought a smelly bundle of moulds wrapped in sacking to the Institute, suggesting that they should be investigated because aboriginal tradition had it that they suppressed infection and promoted healing.

Closer to home, the East Hoathly, East Sussex, agriculturist Thomas Tusser, author of a *Five Hundred Pointes of Good Husbandrie* (1544, 1573), noted that white witches and wise women in Sussex villages used mouldy bread to facilitate the healing of wounds and to treat burns. Thomas Goodyer, the Petersfield botanist, noted in 1627 that wise women and cunning men in Hampshire and West Sussex used a mush of mouldy bread in milk to treat impetigo, cuts, wounds, burns, and all manner of skin infections.

A letter to the *News Chronicle* in 1892 described how:

'In many Sussex farmhouses and cottages the Good Friday bun was allowed to hang suspended from the grimy beams of the kitchen ceiling and there were a number of superstitions attached to it. Foremost among these was the tradition that the mouldy portions removed from time to time and mushed with water were suitable as curative agents for many complaints or disorders and these pseudo-remedies were exploited to treat both humans and cattle' (see **Easter Bun**).

A similar practice was evidently widespread elsewhere in Europe, as witness this account by Dr E.A. Cliffe:

'It was during a visit through Central Europe in 1908 that I came across the fact that almost every farmhouse followed the practice of keeping a mouldy loaf on one of the beams in the kitchen. When I asked the reason for this I was told that this was an old custom and that when any member of the family received an injury such as a cut or a bruise, a thin slice of mouldy bread from the outside of the loaf was cut off, mixed into a paste with water and applied to the wound with a bandage. It was assumed that no infection could result from such a cut.'

Less frequently, reference is also made to the curative virtues of moulds developed on fruit. Here is an account from Mr D.C. McCarthy:

'Many years ago an old aunt of mine (who was 82 years old, and lived in Uckfield), who appeared to be quite learned in 'cures', read one day in a newspaper of Prof Fleming's discovery of penicillin which was described as resulting from research on a mould. My aunt said in her own inimitable way "I had that one before he did". I know that one of her cures was to collect 10-12 oranges and place them somewhere where they could get mouldy as soon as possible. She would then carefully remove the greenish mould and make it into some kind of concoction/defusion/infusion and use it on abscesses, boils, whitlows and other

117

forms of pustule. She would also administer it orally for a great variety of complaints, and all apparently with complete success.'

Even more rarely, reference is given to the therapeutic uses of moulds developed on animal products such as lard. For example, this account forwarded by Mrs Ida Collingwood:

'My grandfather, when I was young and used to stay with him at Lewes (about the early 1920s) and if we had nasty cuts and scabs from falling down, used to get his penknife and scrape the bacon side hung from the ceiling (to be cured), salted and *green*, and put the mouldy fat on a piece of clean linen and grandma used to wrap our knees up and it always cleaned and healed our wounds.'

In a similar vein the following appeared in the *Daily Express* in 1943:

'Mrs Eva Wood is a little scornful of the new wonder drug that has been discovered from mould called penicillin. Her great grandmother, who lived in Petworth, used to collect all the new copper pennies she could, and old copper kettles, smear them with lard and leave them in a damp place. When the mould had formed she would scrape it off into the little boxes and everyone for miles around came to her for the remedy for what ailed them.'

The most detailed account I have seen of the use of moulds in popular medicine is the story of how Mrs Brenda Ward (née Whitnear) was as a child in Brighton cured of a bad case of impetigo by the application of a mould poultice. In the summer of 1926 eight year old Brenda was suffering from severe impetigo, an infection caused by the bacterium *Staphylococcus aureus*. The infection failed to respond to the conventional therapy, so Brenda's family doctor, Dr James Twomey, tried as a last resort what he described as an old Sussex folk remedy. He told Brenda's mother to make some domestic hot water starch into a paste the consistency of lemon curd. The paste was then to be left in the pantry while it developed a mould. On his return, Twomey told Brenda's mother to apply the mouldy starch to the girl's face and use a face mask to keep it in contact with the impetigo crusts. Within a week the impetigo was cured.

The substrates used to grow moulds for use in folk medicine were almost invariably foodstuffs, such as bread, fruit, vegetables, meat, or grains. These substrates tend to become contaminated almost exclusively by species of *Penicillium* and *Aspergillus* which manufacture and release a wide range of bacteriocidal antibiotics, including penicillin.

## OYSTERS

Miss Hilda Petts, born in Manor Road, Selsey in 1913, and at the time of writing living in Albion Road, remembers Selsey when fishing was its chief occupation. Her great-grandfather, a former customs officer from Kent, came to Selsey before 1800 and became a fishmonger. His sons were fishermen, and her father, James, was one until an accident in 1935 ended his career.

Many fisherfolk lived in Albion Road – before her time it was called Fishshops Lane – and as a young girl she ate oysters dredged off Church Norton, where there were also productive winkle beds. 'When my mother had a bad bout of 'flu which was hard to shake off,' she remembers, 'she was advised to eat oysters lightly fried in bacon fat – and that did the trick.'

## PAYMENT BY RESULTS

Among some documents found in the Parish Chest at Cuckfield by the Revd M. Cooper in 1922 was the following Agreement relating to the treatment of a sick parishioner, made between a local apothecary, George Mace, and members

119

of the Parish Vestry responsible for disbursements under the Poor Law (see **Poor Law Medicine**):

## MEMORANDUM

An Agreemt made between we whose names are underwritten all Inhabitants of the parish of Cockfeild and George Mace of Cockfeild Apothecary this day of December 1723.

First We the Inhabitants have agreed to pay George Mace the sum of Four pounds four shillings in case he makes a perfect cure of Thomas Bashfords Legg and Foot before Easter Next. In Case the said George Mace does not make a Cure of the said Thomas Bashfords Legg and Foot before Easter next. Then We agree to pay him Four Pounds and Four Shillings within a yr after He shall have made a perfect Cure of the said Bashfords Legg and Foot. But in case the said Geroge Mace shall make a Perfect Cure of the said T.Bashfords legg and Foot before Easter next and shall have reced the Four pound and four shilings for so doing and the said T. Bashfords Legg and Foot shall happen to grow bad again within a yr of the same Cause then It is agreed that the said Gorge Mace shall repay the said Four pounds Four shillings into some of the parishioners hands for the parish Use

Witness our Hands – Robt Norden Charles Savage Berd Heasman Mich Feild, Churchwardens. Water Gatland William Anscomb, Overseers. George Mace

In the absence of more information on the local context, I don't believe that my interpretation of the significance of this Agreement would be more authoritative than that of anyone else. So far as I am aware, such 'payment by results' Agreements were not common, and certainly not the norm. This one may reflect an unusually strong-minded financially tight Parish Vestry suspicious of the competence and ability to deliver of licensed medics; or a Vestry which felt itself to be in a particularly strong position in its negotiations with an apothecary whose position was weak. May this have been because he was widely viewed as incompetent? or in financial difficulties? or in competition with another local physician for the Poor Law contract?, perhaps a combination of these factors?

## PLAGUE: THREE SUSSEX CURES

Plague was one of the most feared diseases of pre-modern England between its arrival on these shores around the time of the Black Death (1348/9) and its virtual, unexplained, disappearance during the 18th-19th centuries (with a last high in the 1660s with the Great Plague and for twenty or so years after). Though mainly associated with the over populated, insalubrious, rat-infested ports and towns – Rye, Seaford, Lewes and Chichester suffered heavy mortality during each of the great epidemics – it threatened the rural population too, and several Sussex villages were erased from the map during the Black Death. It could be picked up at markets and fairs, and epidemics could spread out, albeit erratically and patchily, into country areas via the agency of fleeing townspeople and/or locals returning from towns.

The earliest remedy for plague I have found in a Sussex source – from little more than a hundred years after the first appearance of plague in England – was noted down in Cowfold's Churchwardens' Accounts during the reign of Edward IV, c 1470-1483:

'Ffor the pestilencie to make a drynke.. Take vedervoy, matfelon and mogworte, solyge, scabyos, avense; make this echelyke myche [take equal quantities?; cut into equal pieces?]; wecke [stir vigorously] 'hem and stampe 'hem, and temper 'hem with stale ale; and get the secke to drynke vi sponysful at ones; and he haf het by tymys [if he takes it in time] hyt shal destroye the coropcion, and sak [save?] the man or the woma[n]'.

Some of the ingredients such as mogworte (mugwort, the common native wormwood *Artemisia vulgaris*) are

121

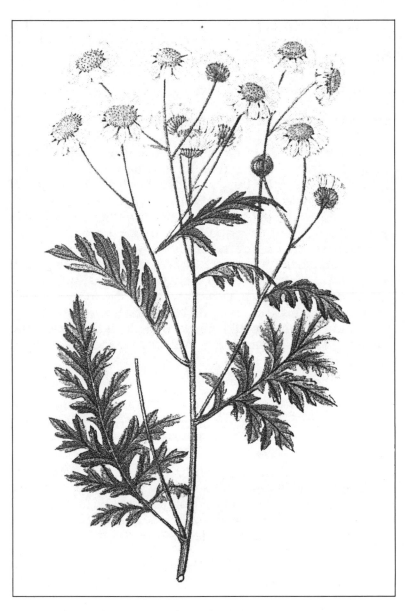

*Feverfew or* Pyrethrum parthenium *from Chaumeton's* Flore Medicale *after an original by Turpin.*

obvious, others less so. Vedervoy, or featherfoy, as it was still known in Sussex until well into the 20th century, is the feverfew – the fever foe or quasi *fugans febre* or fever fugue for putting fevers to flight – formerly grown in every physic and many cottage gardens and widely used, and at least partly effective, against fevers ranging from plague and agues (malaria) to common 'flu, and also for headaches and as an emmenagogue (menstruation aid). The herb is reckoned as of great virtue by the shepherd in *The Play of the Shepherds*, one of the Chester Plays:

'Here be more erbes I tell it to you,/I shall reckon them on a rooe,/Fynter fanter and *fetter foe*,/And also perye wyrtle.'

Matfelon, or 'Materfilon, otherwise Matrefillon' as it appears in Lovell's *Pambotanologia*, is the black knapweed, a decoction of which was used as a tonic in rural Sussex into recent times. Avense is herb bennet or avens. Solyge could be smallage, the wild celery, or ploughman's spikenard (Gerard's 'Sellage'), or the sundew *Rosa Solis* or sollyge, widely used in plague preparations in the 15th and 16th centuries.

Scabyos could be the obvious scabious, the scabies herb widely used to consume plague buttons; or its relative the devil's bit scabious *Succisa pratensis*, a traditional plague and fever herb formerly called scabious in many regions; or any of several other herbs known locally as scabious because they were deemed useful against scabies.

The latest plague cure I have found in a Sussex source is in a small octavo volume published by the Revd William Turner in 1685, not long after the Great Plague:

'The plague drink: Take three quarters of Malaga sack and boil therein a handful of blue, until one part be wasted. Then strain it and set it on the fire again and put into it a pennyworth of long pepper, half an oz of ginger, and a quarter of an oz of nutmegs, all beaten up together. After it has been boiled a little time add to it a pennyworth of treacle and a quarter of a pint of Angelica water. Keep this by you, as above all wordly treasures. Take it warm always, both evening and morning – a spoonful or two, if you be already infected – and sweat yourself well with it. But if you be not infected a spoonful once a day is sufficient. In all the Plague have trust in God. And then, by using the above drink, neither man nor woman, neither stripling nor child labouring under the dire disease can infect you with it.'

In a diary entry dated the 24th May 1665, during the Great Plague,the Revd John Allin, puritan Vicar of Rye, alchemist, astrologer, merchant and speculator, notes that 'many persons here wear amulets against plague made of the poison of toads which upon infection raise a blister which a plaister heals, and so they are cured.'

## PLAGUE STONE

In September 1930 Sussex author Jane Wolseley visited an old house called Scrag Oak in the parish of Wadhurst, which was then for sale. In the garden on the west side was a large grey stone which had been moved from another position on the property, and was locally designated as a plague stone. It was a block some three feet square, slightly irregular in shape, and the centre had been hollowed out to form a deep basin, in one corner of which there appeared to be a small opening to allow any excess of liquid to flow away.

The purpose of such stones – mentioned by Defoe in his *History of the Plague* [comprising his *Journal of the Plague Year* and *Due Preparations for the Plague*] – was to enable those afflicted with the plague, or who had been exposed to contagion, to get provisions by placing coins in the basin which for disinfecting purposes was filled with vinegar. The unaffected person placed provisions on the wide ledge of the stone, took the coins and then retired.

# POOR LAW MEDICINE

'Rattle his bones, over the stones
He's only a pauper whom nobody owns'

From the 16th to early 20th centuries, a quarter to a third of the population could expect to come to this, a solitary burial as a vagrant or from the workhouse, poor law hospital, or madhouse.

Begging was universal – beggars at the door, outside the churches, in the market place and wandering along the roads. Beyond the inner circle of those who made up respectable society were the vast and troubling army of unmentionables: beggars, paupers, half-starved cottagers, *les gens du néant*; people born to destitution, or who had been forced to go under, obliged to take to the roads as beggars or to throw themselves on the not always gentle mercies of the community.

Of course, beggars and the poor had been there in the Middle Ages. But they had been a structural, accepted part of the medieval system, succoured and supported, if scarcely cosseted, by the all-embracing charity of the Church and by more or less morally and socially obligatory private charity.

From about 1500 onwards, their numbers began to increase alarmingly – as a result of the traumatic social and economic changes then occurring – and their place in a more individualistic, materialistic and market-oriented society had become problematical. From 1563-1601 a series of Acts of Parliament laid down the guidelines for dealing with poverty, unemployment, and conditions of employment. These shaped the 'Poor Law', a system which, with only minor modifications and tinkering along the way, was to regulate treatment of the poor, and their access to licensed medical treatment, for some 400 years, into the early 20th century.

The measures ranged from savage laws against vagrants and beggars, the 'undeserving poor' (a definition born of, and symptomatic of, the new age) – which did nothing to stem the inexorable rise in their numbers – to more or less ambiguous charitable and welfare measures. These included the construction and running of almshouses, poorhouses/workhouses and poor law hospitals and support, and limited provision of medical care for the 'deserving' sick, destitute and elderly, all paid for out of a 'Poor Rate' which was assessed, levied and administered at a local level parish by parish. They were ambiguous because they might be regarded simultaneously as hard-headed measures to reduce vagrancy, keep the lid on social unrest, and put the poor to work at minimum cost, but also as a continuation of the medieval tradition, acts of Christian charity and communal solidarity towards the least fortunate.

Be that as it may, under the Poor Law system parishes did make more or less generous or grudging provision for the medical care of paupers in their poor and alms houses and for some of those in the community at large too poor to afford medical treatment.

Fascinating insights into the world of the Poor Law and Poor Law medicine have come from Michael Gowler's analysis of poor relief in Bognor between 1790 and 1840. I shall draw heavily on his study, while bringing in complementary material from other Sussex sources. At this time the Sutton Union Poorhouse served some 15-16 parishes including Southbersted to which Bognor at that time belonged. The poorhouse was supported by the Poor Rate levied in the member parishes.

Relief of the poor had always been in the hands of the Church and the Church Vestry was the body used for that purpose. It consisted of men elected from the parish to run the affairs of the parish, and was chaired by the vicar or incumbent of the time. The elected members were well-to-do parishioners: gentlemen, farmers, professionals, tradesmen. They met at regular intervals in the parish church.

Out of their number they elected each year two church-wardens, two Overseers of the Poor and a Guardian of the Poor. The overseers were responsible for the assessment and collection of the Poor Rate, within the very loose guidelines provided by successive Acts of Parliament (the rules only being tightened and made explicit in the Poor Law

Amendment Act of 1834). The Guardian was the relieving officer. His main duty was to relieve the poor using monies collected in Poor Tax: to make the parish's contribution to the running of its own or a Union's poorhouse, and to disburse monies for the medical treatment and general relief of the poor in his parish. He was a paid official, the others were not.

Until the 1834 Act, the collection and disbursement of Poor Rate monies was subject only to control and supervision by the Parish Vestry and, in theory, though seldom in practice, by the justices of the peace. The inevitable result was that the system might be benevolent or cruel, generous or niggardly, honest or corrupt, efficient or slipshod and wasteful as the local officers and local public opinion decided. At its best, the system provided generous help for the poor and basic medical treatment for the sick poor; helped redistribute income; and provided local employment (for those nursing the sick, providing services, etc). At its worst, Poor Rate monies levied on the many went not to the relief of the poor and sick but via multiple routes into the pockets of the minority who controlled and administered the system. After the 1834 Act, Poor Law was still paid out of local rates, but the parishes were obligatorily grouped together into unions of parishes, each with its own local board of governors elected *ad hoc*. These boards and their accounts were tightly supervised by a central Board of Commissioners sitting in London.

Each year a local surgeon or apothecary was appointed to care for the paupers in the poorhouse and in the parishes of the Union, or individual parish. He received a salary which covered visits and medicines. He received extra fees for emergencies, such as fractures, vagrants, difficult pregnancies etc. Throughout much of this time, the salary paid by the Sutton Union was £35 pa. When there was more than one surgeon or apothecary in a Poor Law area, they might be appointed in alternate years, or for alternating three month periods. Near the beginning of the period the tendency was to appoint surgeons and/or apothecaries. By the early 19th century the tendency was to appoint only surgeons, except in areas where there were no surgeons/physicians and an apothecary was the only licensed practitioner: an indication of a change in the function of apothecaries, from medical generalists particularly skilled in the preparation and prescription of drugs to prescribing pharmacists with ancillary medical skills.

On many occasions the Southbersted surgeons prescribed the drinking of port wine or porter to fortify patients. These 'medicines' were supplied by local innkeepers. There is one invoice from Joseph Leal of West Street dated 1834, requesting payment of £1.10s for supplying porter to Mrs Waller's daughter over a period of eight months. At 2s per gallon, this works out at 240 days at half a pint a day, which appears to have been the daily ration for girls.

The surgeon also had authority to order meat (usually mutton) to aid the diet of the sick. This was supplied by local butchers who sent their bills to the Parish Vestry for payment.

On the nursing side, there seems to have been over the years a good supply of women available to nurse the sick and attend to pregnant women at their lying-in. If the patients were paupers, the parish paid the women for their services. In long-term cases, they sometimes took turns to nurse. Payment varied between 3/6d and 5s per week, sometimes with tea and sugar thrown in – or even a decidedly liberal ration of gin.

Over the years, there were many cases of insanity, which usually meant special nursing care on a 24-hour basis and then an examination and commitment to an asylum to undergo the barbarically uncomprehending treatment meted out to the mentally deranged in those days. The institution used by the Sutton Union was the infamous madhouse at Bethnal Green under the management of Dr Warburton and his colleagues.

Payments under these account heads included surgeons's fees, transport expenses for patient and escort to London, regular payments for maintenance and treatment of the patient while in the asylum and a fee to a doctor to make an annual visit to examine and report on his or her condition.

Sometimes vagrants fell ill while within the parish boundary and had to be cared for. They were usually installed in one of the inns and tended by local women. Payments were then made to the innkeeper for board and lodgings, to the nurse and to the patient, when sufficiently recovered, to get him or her back on the road. See also **Sedlescombe, A 17th century Doctor's Bill.**

# RABBITS

In a short 'Folklore Note' published in 1935 (*Sussex County Magazine*, 9,698), H.S. Toms writes:

'Turning to another side of folklore in which both rabbits and hares are beneficient or connected with good fortune, there is the interesting belief that the brain of either animal should be cooked as nutriment for soothing troublesome or craving infants. This is a specific known in Dorset, and also in Sussex; for the writer is reminded that rabbit brains were recommended for use on his small boy at Brighton, in May 1907 (by a charwoman) and also that the specific was effective.'

There seem to be late lingering memories of two ancient beliefs here. The first is 'sympathetic magic': that by ingesting the flesh (and notably the brain) of an animal one might ingest and assimilate its qualities. In primitive tribes warriors ate the brains of lions in the belief that this would make them more courageous (and refrained from eating tortoise flesh because this would render them slow of wit and foot). Similarly, eating the brains of docile rabbits could be expected to make a troublesome infant less turbulent and more docile (in effect, it would assimilate the rabbit's docility which would cancel out its own inner turbulence).

The same idea was at work in the old Sussex custom of feeding dove's flesh to people suffering from fever (the legendary coolness, docility and gentleness of the dove counteracting and cancelling out the heat and turbulence of the fever).

The second, overlapping, belief is the Roman to early modern Theory of the Humours, whereby ill health or disturbed behaviour were traceable to imbalances between the 'Four Humours' or 'Qualities': here using the assimilated qualities of the docile, non-choleric rabbit to cancel out an excess of 'Choler'.

For other examples of 'sympathetic magic', see **Badger; Hedgehog, Swallows;** for more on the Four Humours, see **Leech-catcher**.


## Runs of the Lights

Bizarre and ineffectual cures had by no means died out in the early 20th century. In a letter to the *Sussex County Magazine* in 1935, Dr L.B. Richardson of Hove wrote:

'The following occurred in my practice some thirty years ago. A very buxom young woman went for a drive with her young man, intending to go to Lewes, but opposite the old Toll Gate at Falmer the dog-cart was overthrown and she was carried into the Toll Gate cottage, where the woman promptly diagnosed her complaint as "Runs of the Lights" [lungs].

'She then proceeded to "sink them". From a corner cupboard she produced an egg-cup, filled it with gunshot and made the young woman swallow it!

'This she told me next morning.'


## Scurvy, scurvy grass and samphire

Scurvy, now known to be a consequence of Vitamin C deficiency, was a widespread killer disease in 16th-18th century

Sussex. A high proportion of the population suffered from this distressing condition, and some died.

> Scurvy was a 'filthie, lothsome, heavie and dull disease [in which] the gums are loosed, swolne and exulcerate; the mouth grievously stinking; the thighes and legs withall veerie often full of blewe spots, not much unlike those that come of bruises; the face and the rest of the body is often times of a pale colour; and the feet is swolne as in the dropsie.'

At first encounter, the prevalence of scurvy in all sections of the population may seem surprising (for an account of one sufferer see **Charlatans: Dr Flugger**). After all, Sussex was profoundly rural. Most of the population lived on farms or in hamlets or villages, or in small towns opening on to the countryside, with easy access to cultivated fruits and vegetables and the riches of Nature's larder. Even in larger towns such as Chichester, Horsham, Lewes and Rye people were never more than a few hundred yards from open countryside, and had the benefit of important markets. We like to imagine the people of olden time Sussex as eating a diet that was healthier and more natural than ours. A disease of calcium deficiency, rickets in the urban poor we can understand, because dairy products, available to all but the most indigent in rural areas, were scarcer and more expensive by the time they got to town; it is less easy to comprehend the prevalence, in rural as well as urban Sussex, of a deficiency disease associated with a diet poor in fresh fruit and vegetables.

Of course, some people did eat vegetables and fruit, from pleasure or necessity. But multiple lines of evidence – from menus, household account books, diaries etc – show that when they had the means many people ate almost exclusively meat, potted meats, game, fish, pies, cheeses, and puddings and sweetmeats of every kind, almost eliminating vegetables from their diet. The archetypal 17th/18th century Englishman was a carnivore with a sweet tooth who had little affection for fresh vegetables, which is one reason why one finds well-off people coming down with scurvy.

131

When people did eat vegetables (from necessity, sometimes for pleasure) or fruit (for pleasure), they still weren't guaranteed an adequate year-long intake of Vitamin C. For a start, the almost universal custom was to boil vegetables to destruction, certainly to the point where most of their Vitamin C was destroyed – not because people were poor cooks, but because vegetables were tougher (if more flavoursome) than today, and because by the time they got to their 30s and 40s and beyond most people had decayed teeth or had lost most of them (a combination of poor oral hygiene and the traditional English love of sweetmeats). Furthermore, people consumed prodigious quantities of salted and smoked foods and drank far more alcohol than modern Englishmen and women: dietary factors which destroy, or inhibit the uptake and deployment of, Vitamin C.

Above all, we too easily forget that vegetables and fruits were seasonal. From October or November through to April there were next to no fresh fruits or vegetables, cultivated or wild, to be had – no local produce and, except for the rich, no imported exotica such as oranges or lemons. For six months of the year the only sources of Vitamin C were keeping fruits such as apples (not rich in Vitamin C anyway) and vegetables such as onions (potatoes were not yet a major item of diet). And even during the natural growing season, cold wet weather and/or destruction by pests could – and frequently did – lead to crop failures and a prolonged dearth of local produce which, because of the state of the roads and the high cost and slow speed of transport, couldn't be compensated by imports from unaffected regions or countries.

The standard physicians' treatment for scurvy from the 16th to late 18th centuries involved the administration of sulphuric acid, on the grounds that scurvy was an 'alkaline' disease. This helps to explain why so many people were wary of physicians, and turned to self-help, cunning women or quacks to cure their ills.

But while an explicit connection between scurvy and a diet poor in fruit and vegetables had yet to be made, there was an undercurrent of awareness that the disease could be treated by herbal/dietary methods.

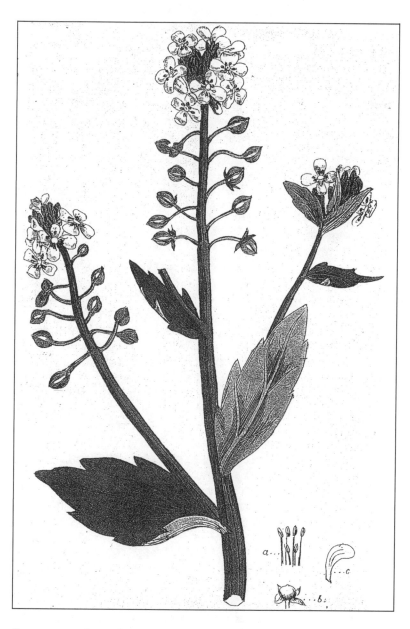

*Scurvy grass from* Flora Medica, *1829.*

One herb recognised as a powerful anti-scorbutic was 'sampher' – samphire – which used to grow at many localities on the then wild and undeveloped Sussex coast. It was collected on a commercial scale, and sold by apothecaries and herb women and at markets. From evidence in documents such as the Dacre household accounts, we know that some wealthy 17th century landowners sent their retainers to coastal towns such as Eastbourne to collect or buy samphire in bulk, to make the household scurvy-free through the winter.

A second herb appreciated for its efficacy against scurvy was, as its name implies, scurvy grass. According to Pliny, the legionnaires of Germanicus Caius, in his campaign across the Rhine, were taught the use of it by the Frisians and rescued from a scurvy-like disease.

Scurvy grass came in two varieties. *Cochlearia officinalis* – *officinalis* being the epithet of the *officina*, the apothecary's shop, hence of plants used in medicine – was an introducee grown in physic and cottage gardens for personal use and for sale to apothecaries. But the cultivated form does not grow prolifically and could not be cultivated on a scale appropriate to the demand, hence supplies were supplemented by collecting the native *C.anglica*, with its narrower, less rounded leaves, which could not be cultivated but grew locally on the marshes of the Thames Estuary and along the Kent and Sussex coasts from Romney Marsh to Eastbourne and from Portslade to Chichester Harbour.

Scurvy grass medicine, in which the unpleasant taste of the herb was disguised with spices and saffron, was popular in the 1600s; and was doubtless familiar to the Dacres of Herstmonceux, whose retainers bought scurvy grass at Eastbourne in the 1640s. Anthony à Wood has described how in the 1650s there was a fashion for a scurvy grass drink in the mornings, like our glass of orange juice. Early in the 19th century, scurvy grass sandwiches were eaten, and 'spring juices' were concocted from scurvy grass, watercress and Seville oranges. It was the pleasanter watercress and lime juice which finally put the older remedy out of fashion.

A couple of questions intrude themselves here. First, why

did so many wealthy people submit to the sulphuric acid torture imposed by their physicians when a gentler, more effective treatment was, apparently, quite well known and accessible to those with reasonable means? Answer have I none, but it must have had something to do with the prestige and (challenged, but not negligible) intellectual authority of physicians basing their science on ancient authorities aureoled with glory such as Hippocrates and Galen and/or the most up to date and fashionable, if often fallacious, scientific theories.

The second question is easier. Why did so many people in 17th and 18th century Sussex endure the horrors of scurvy when a herbal remedy was known (perhaps not to everyone, but widely) and available? The answer seems to be that the supply of cultivated scurvy grass was limited, and wild sampher and scurvy grass only occurred at coastal sites, which grew progressively fewer as a result of over-exploitation and, in the 18th century, the mushrooming growth of coastal resorts such as Eastbourne, Hove, Worthing, Littlehampton, and Bognor Regis. Much of this limited supply was used by local people along the coast, or bought up by the Navy (though it could never get enough to defeat scurvy at sea), by wealthy households such as the Dacres, and by middlemen supplying apothecaries. In areas of Sussex away from the coast scurvy grass did not get through to local markets and was only available from apothecaries (and, perhaps, travelling quacks such as Dr Flugger?) in the form of pills and potions to expensive for most pockets.


## SEDLESCOMBE, A 17TH CENTURY DOCTOR'S BILL

In 1930 Mr N.T. Ticehurst of St Leonards came across the following account while sorting through miscellaneous documents in the parish chest at Sedlescombe. The account is for medical expenditure on the poor under the Poor Law (see **Poor Law Medicine**).

| 'Aprill ye 11th: 89 | li. | s. | d |
|---|---|---|---|
| A Clister for ye Maide | 00 | 00 | 08 |
| A Paralytic deobstructive gargle ye boy | 00 | 01 | 06 |
| Bleeding him under the tongue | 00 | 01 | 00 |
| A Blister for ye Maides necke | 00 | 00 | 08 |
| A Cordiall Coroberateing Apozem for them | 00 | 02 | 08 |
| A Cordiall Cephalic Jelepe for them | 00 | 01 | 06 |
| A strengtheninge Restringent Electuary ye maide | 00 | 01 | 06 |
| Four Narcotic Pills | 00 | 00 | 06 |
| A Paralytic Electuary ye Boy | 00 | 01 | 06 |
| Twelue Hypnotic Pills | 00 | 01 | 00 |
| Cordiall strengtheninge Ingredients for 3 quarts of Liquor | 00 | 01 | 06 |
| More of the Same | 00 | 01 | 06 |
| A strengthening Apertiue Electuary | 00 | 01 | 08 |
| A Cathartic Electuary ye girle for severall doses | 00 | 01 | 06 |
| | 00 | 18 | 08 |
| ffor Care and visites | 00 | 06 | 00 |
| Totall summe | 01 | 04 | 08 |

May ye 6th: 89

Recd of Jon Huckstepe Ouerseare the sume of one pound four shillings and eight pence being in full of this Bill for Phisicke administd to Ann Blatcher and John Henlly of the parish of Sedlescombe. Recd me Jon Martin 1 li 4s 8d'

Apozem – decoction or infusion.
Blister – anything applied to raise a blister.
Cathartic – cleansing, purging.
Cephalic – for curing or relieving disorders of the head.
Clister – rectal injection, enema or suppository; the syringe used in the injection or its contents; also in the 16th and 17th centuries a popular contemptuous name for a medical practitioner.
Cordiall – invigorating, or stimulating to the circulation.
Cor(r)oberating – strengthening, fortifying, invigorating.

Electuary – a medicinal conserve or paste, consisting of a powder or other ingredient mixed with honey or syrup.

Hypnotic/Narcotic – soporific, sleep-inducing.

Julepe – a liquid sweetened with honey or syrup and used as a vehicle for a medicine.

Paralytic – any medicine inducing paralysis: anaesthetic and/or pain-killing.

Restringent – astringent, binding, tending to restrain the action of the bowels (or a styptic, when applied externally).

## SHREW, SHREW ASH AND SHREW HAZEL

In former times, shrews were widely believed to have a poisonous bite. Folklore has many references to the toxicity of shrews, to people killed and livestock lamed or killed by the biting, even the baleful nocturnal breathing, or the 'running' of shrews. For example, this in the Revd Edward Topsell's splendid *Historie of Foure-Footed Beastes and Serpents: Describing at Large their True and Lively Figure, their Several Names, Conditions, Kinds, Virtues (both Natural and Medicinal), Countries of their Breed, their Love and Hatred of Mankinde, and the Wonderful Work of God in Their Creation, Preservation, and Destruction. Interwoven with Curious Variety of Historical Narrations out of Scriptures, Fathers, Philosophers, Physicians and Poets; Illustrated with Divers Hieroglypicks and Emblems: both Pleasant and Profitable for Students in all Faculties and Professions*, (1607):

'It is a ravening Beast, feyning itself gentle and tame, but, being touched, it biteth deep and poysoneth deadly. There is nothing which do more apparently explain and shew the biting of a Shrew than a certain vehement pain and grief in the creature which is so bitten, as also a pricking over the whole body, with an inflammation or burning heat going around the place, and a fiery redness therein, in which a black push or like swelling with a watery matter and filthy corrupcion doth arise until all parts of the body which do

137

joyn unto it seem black and blew with a marvellous great pain, anguish, and grief which proceedeth and ariseth from the same'

Now recent research has shown that common and, to a greater degree, water shrews do have a poisonous bite which they use to paralyse or kill worms, cockroaches, newts and similar small creatures. But as shrews seldom have the opportunity to bite people and would be incapable of biting through the thick hide of cows or horses, and as it is doubtful that any successful bites would have baleful consequences (the venom is relatively weak compared with say, snake venom, and the quantity injected small), it seems probable that the age-old belief in the poisonous bite of shrews is a myth which happens, quite by chance, to overlap with the truth. The association of shrews and poison probably has its origins in the foully poisonous odour of the shrew which deters predators.

One remedy for shrew-bite (or rather for conditions in man and beast – aches, pains, mysterious rashes, lameness – attributed to the nocturnal running or biting of shrews) involved the use of a shrew ash into which a shrew had been walled alive. Several accounts of shrew ashes or other shrew trees in Sussex and its immediately adjoining regions have come down to us, the best known being in Gilbert White's *The Natural History and Antiquities of Selborne* (1789):

'At the south corner of the Plestor, or area near the church, there stood about 20 years ago a very old, grotesque, hollow pollard ash which for ages had been looked on with no small veneration as a shrew ash. Now a shrew ash is an ash whose twigs, when gently applied to the limbs of cattle, will immediately relieve the pain which a beast suffers from the running of a shrew mouse over the part affected; for it is supposed that a shrew mouse is of so baleful and deleterious a nature that wherever it creeps over a beast, be it horse, cow, or sheep, the suffering animal is afflicted with cruel anguish and threatened with the loss of the use of the limb. Against this accident, to which they are continually liable, our prudent forefathers always kept a shrew ash at hand, which once medicated would maintain its virtues for ever.'

And here is a fuller, less familiar account in the Revd Gordon's *History and Natural History of Harting*, 1877:

'A shrew gives out such a rank unpleasant odour that, although a cat will readily kill it, we have never heard of a cat eating one. The odour is not unlike a compound of garlic and musk and may, not improbably, have given rise to the popular belief that the shrew is venomous. Not only is its bite considered by its fellow parishioners to be capable of producing very serious consequences to man and his domestic animals, but even simple contact with any part of the body is dreadful. Fortunately for the present and future generations, our earlier naturalists have left us simple instructions for the successful treatment of all genuine cases of shrew bite – a live shrew, an auger, a plug of wood, and a sound growing ash tree are all that is required for the purpose; a hole is bored in the body of the tree, the poor shrew securely plugged in it, and from that moment the branches and leaves of the 'shrew ash' acquire the wonderful property of neutralizing the venom of any number of shrews! Will it be needful to add that the bite of this little animal is perfectly harmless to man!'

And here is a third account, this time of a shrew-hazel, from Mr H. Toms in *Sussex Notes and Queries*:

'In this connection Mr B. Morris (Hon. Sec. of the Newhaven Literary and Debating Society) tells me that "when out for a walk with other boys and a form master at Ardingly in 1883, I saw in a spinney what appeared to be a sedge-warbler's nest. Next day I and another lad broke bounds to investigate this 'nest' and found it to be a stoutish hazel twig cut off short with a curious lump on it. The stick had been split, and in the split something inserted. The whole was covered with clay and subsequently bound round with straw or twisted hay which gave the lump the appearance of a nest. We opened it and found a putrid shrew mouse inside, the ends of the split stick having been drawn together at the top before plastering with clay." The owner of the land, a typical small farmer, was subsequently interviewed but he would not admit any knowledge of the matter personally; though he said that his parents had been firm believers in the efficacy of the practice as a cure for ailing cattle which had probably been bitten or run over by a shrew.'

'The touch of an ashen bough causeth a giddiness in the viper's head', writes Tomas Nashe in *Pierce Penniless*. The use of an ash, above all other trees, against the biting or running of shrews was not arbitrary, but the continuation of a tradition dating back to Graeco-Roman times. The ash was *the* tree against evil and poison. Here, for example, is Gerard (1597):

'The leaves of this tree are of so great a virtue against serpents, so that the serpents dare not be so bolde as to touch the morning and evening shaddowes of the tree, but shunneth them a farre off.'

In Ireland, ash wood was burned to banish the Devil. And here is John Lightfoot in his *Flora Scotica* (1777):

'In many parts of the Highlands, at the birth of a child, the nurse or midwife, for what motive I know not, puts one end of a green stick of this tree into the fire and, while it is burning, receives into a spoon the syrup or juice which oozes out of the other end, and administers this as the first spoonful of liquor to the newborn baby.'

It was a way of giving the child the strength of the ash and protecting it from pixies and goblins.

As to why ash was *the* tree against poison and evil, we can only guess. The two key points may be, first, that it has one of the strongest and most elastic timbers; hence was

140

considered to be highly resistant to, or the antithesis of, corruption, poison, and decay. It was thus able both to repel the powers of evil and their expression in poison, and to convey, by sympathetic magic, some of its resistance to evil to those who established a contact with it by imbibing preparations made from ash, etc. For an important and widespread application of the ash in the cure of childhood hernias, involving sympathetic magic and the strength and elastic properties of the ash, see **Trees**.

Second, lightning runs to the ash – 'Avoid the ash, it courts the flash'. A reminder that, like the oak ('Avoid an oak, it courts the stroke'), it was a tree of power favoured of, and sacred to, the Ancient Greek sky and thunder gods such as Zeus and his Roman successor Jupiter. The ash was a tree of the sky gods hostile and antithetical to the chthonic – earth or subterranean divinities – many of whom, like Dionysius, were snake gods, and Hecate and other gods and goddesses of the underworld who increasingly came to be associated with Hell and the powers of Evil.

# SLUGS

'Here is an old Sussex remedy given to my father when a lad (about 80 years ago) by an old woman. To cure a whitlow – Place a large black slug on a piece of clean rag and stick it all over with a needle. Wrap the affected finger in the rag.'

M. Chapman, East Grinstead

(for another cure of whitlows see **Moulds**).

In a once-popular Sussex cure for warts a large slug was impaled on a thorn and as the slug shrivelled and died the wart slowly declined in size until it finally disappeared. Some said that the slug, which in Sussex was usually the all-black or orange *Arion ater*, should first be rubbed on to the excrescence – thus establishing some sort of magical connection between the destiny of the slug and that of the wart – and its slime allowed to dry.

## SMALLPOX

Smallpox was the disease that came from nowhere to bring dread and horror into the lives of our ancestors in the 17th, 18th and 19th centuries. The 'white plague' was far more terrible than the 'black' plague it slowly replaced, because whereas the black plague was intermittent and epidemic – largely confined, except in its very worst epidemics, to the towns; and relatively quiet for long periods – smallpox was there all the time, all around one, in the lives of rich and poor, everywhere in town and countryside. It was a disease which usually killed, terribly. When it didn't kill, its survivors were hideously disfigured.

Little known before the reign of Elizabeth I, it began to take hold during that of the first James. Its incidence increased throughout the 17th century and it was *the* killer disease throughout the 18th and into the early/mid 19th centuries.

The Parish Registers of Sussex have many entries reflecting the terrible mortality it inflicted, like this from the Bosham Register for 1741: 'Buried in this and the foregoing year about 16 of the small pox. Richard Lawson, Vicar'. All the 18th century Sussex diarists – for example, the Stapleys and Marchants – make repeated references to family, friends or neighbours – often the healthy young, and the well-off, not just indigents, infants or the old – falling victim to smallpox.

Something of the horror associated with smallpox can be gauged from this passage in R.F. Whistler's memoir on the *Life of the Revd Whistler of Hastings in the 18th and 19th centuries*:

'The following circumstances will serve to show the extreme care that should be taken in order that any disturbance of the bodies of those who have died of smallpox may be carefully avoided. Many years after the

142

above date [1731], and during the absence of the sexton, there was occasion for the burial of a stranger in All Saints [Hastings] churchyard. An apparently vacant spot was soon found by the sexton's substitute who, on disturbing the soil, found that the ground had been previously used, and that several bodies had already been interred there. These were the remains of those who had died of small-pox at the time mentioned. But a few days passed before the symptoms of the infection developed themselves in this unfortunate grave-digger, who sickened and died a victim to this most malignant disease.'

This horror was incarnated in the dreadful and dreaded pesthouses which came to exist beyond the bounds of most large towns in Sussex and throughout the countryside, where they usually served a union of parishes. Here smallpox victims were confined like lepers away from contact with the outside world, fed by packages introduced through windows on the ends of poles, and/or cared for by often hideously disfigured people who had survived the infection and were presumed immune. Old documents attest to the existence of the pesthouses and there are many passing references to them in contemporary sources – for example, a mention of the Chichester Pest House in **Typhoid** – but the precise locations of many are still uncertain because they have been lost to local memory, a collective amnesia which may reflect the horror they induced.

From the early 18th century, medicine did come up with a response of a kind to smallpox, in the form of inoculation, though whether it had much effect on the incidence of the malady is debatable.

Inoculation or 'variolation' was carried out by inoculating material from persons suffering from mild varieties of smallpox, in order to induce a benign form of the disease and thus immunize the patient against the development of more severe forms. In 1718 Lady Mary Wortley Montagu had her son inoculated. In 1722 two of the British royal family were inoculated and from the 1740s to 90s the practice of inoculation became widespread, despite the risks.

For risks there were. Although inoculation was an innovative daring medical advance which could impart immunity, many inoculees developed more severe forms of the disease and were disfigured for life or died. Paul Dunvan, in his *History of Lewes and Brighthelmstone*, 1795, recorded that of 2,113 people inoculated in a mass inoculation in that area 'no more than 50' died – a death rate of one person in 43, with other sources indicating rates ranging from one in five to one in 150 (the efficacy and risks of the treatment depending greatly on the skill, and integrity, of the doctor in choosing material for inoculation).

Here's an extract from Spershott's *Memoirs of 18th Century Chichester*, 1740:

'Inoculation for the Small Pox, which was first brought into England from Turkey in 1724, was now first practised in Chichester, my Self the 3rd Person that came under the Operation: about 300 were inoculated of which I think 3 or 4 died'. [In fact, inoculation had been suggested by Dr Timoni to the Royal Society in 1713; and was introduced from Turkey by Lady Mary Wortley Montagu in 1717/18].

But the attractions of taking a one-off risk and, hopefully, becoming immune to this terrible disease for life were so great that inoculation became immensely popular. Doctors carried out mass inoculations in poorhouses, paid for under the Poor Rate; and made considerable profits carrying out great public inoculations. For example, here is a Ditchling surgeon's advertisement dated 1 September 1760:

'Cooper Sampson, Surgeon of Ditchling, gives Notice, that he begins to inoculate as usual, upon Ditchling Common, the Beginning of this Instant, September, and intends to continue this Practice till June next, at Five Guineas each Person, he finding all manner of Necessaries (Airing included). All persons who intend to come under his care are desired to give him previous Notice, and they shall have directions how to proceed and may count upon constant Attention, careful Nursing, and civil Treatment. He is also ready to wait upon Gentlemen, Ladies, or others, and inoculate any of their Families at their own Habitations, upon very reasonable Terms. He likewise takes in any Person that may fail in the natural way, at six hrs warning at all Times in the Year at Six Guineas and a Half, they paying down Four Guineas at their first Entrance, the rest at going off.'

Many doctors and surgeons set up private smallpox clinics which in many respects were the first private hospitals. Following inoculation, the sons and daughters of the well-to-do could endure their (presumably) attenuated bout of smallpox and recuperate in comfortable rural surroundings – usually in a large isolated house out in the countryside – where they could receive follow-up treatment and parcels, messages or waves from their families.

In 1749, for example, Jane and Mary Collier, daughters of John Collier, five times Mayor of Hastings, spent six months at Northiam at the private inoculation establishment started at this time by Dr Frewen; from whence Mary wrote the following letter to her mother giving something of the flavour of these establishments and the lives of their inmates:

'Honr'd Madam　　　　　　　　　At Doctor Frewen's
　　　　　　　　　　　　　Northiam March ye 30th 1749
I received your letter yesterday and think Hastings by all accounts must have been very Gay this week, with this Grand Wedding. I have at ye same time a long letter from Miss Cruttendon. She sent us some Wedding Cake; so that now we have had 2 sorts to Try ye virtue of it in Dreams but to own ye truth we have not laid any of it yet; but do all intend to do it to night if we don't forget it, just to Try what effect it will have upon us, as they have been so good as to send it to us. Ye business of Inoculation goes on Briskly for there are Six to come into this House ye Day that we go out of it, who are now at Peas marsh. I have this

minute recd a letter of congratulations from my uncle Cranston, but realy ye Bottom of his letter has quite given us ye vapours, with his account of ye Earthquake ye other morning in London sure it is a very odd Thing and quite new in These parts but I Think our Climate is quite altered I'm sure tis not so Cold as it used to be, and I fancy that must be ye reason of it, I find by Miss Morland that our vails [tips] to ye nurses and other Servants will amount to a pretty deal and I imagine you will have us do as other people do in that Case, I beg you will give our Duty to my Papa etc.

Your most Dutifull Daughter M. Collier

PS if ye please, when you send the Things to Rye, I should be glad of my worked Ruffle's one of my rows of Falls Curles with my paper Broad ribbons all of which are in my right Hand Draws'.

That Dr Frewen's competence to inoculate was not universally accepted is suggested by this letter from Uncle Cranston to John Collier on 30 June 1749: 'I heartily pray success may attend my nieces under the inoculation, which I should have been glad to have been done at any place other than Northiam.'

And here are some entries from the diary of John Baker, a solicitor of the Inner Temple, who at 59 years of age came with his wife to reside at Horsham, in the house which is now called Horsham Park:

'April 12 1774. This afternoon Jenny Wisdom, Becky, Betty, Kitchen, Nancy went to Dr Lindfield's.

14. Walked out afternoon. Meant to go to see people at Dr L's house, where they are. He takes in Mr Reid's [a Horsham surgeon] inoculated people, but wind so keen turned back.

15. Went out in Chaise with Fanny and Molly Maul to Dr L's house beyond Champion's Windmill. Chaise stood

about 30 yds from house, but saw all our 7 pox folk. Betty came nr chariot.

19. After dinner Charles went out to Dr L's, said Ned had about 30 pustules small pox, his daughter Jenny 9 or 10, all come out.

20. A little before 7, all the 7 smallpox people came to outside poles, where this morning gave them warm punch and jelly.

21. Walked to Dr L's and saw all the smallpox folk. Sent them at night 2 bottles of punch with the jellies. Charles gave it to William Wiston in at the window (they would not let him come in), for them to eat and drink going to bed.

27. *Soir* came Mr Reid, agreed to take home all the inoculees next Tuesday, and inoculate other 5 next Sunday. He said if they first caught it in the natural way, and were inoculated 3 or 4 days after, the latter would defeat the former, and take place entirely.'

In 1796 Jenner discovered the process of vaccination, whereby vaccination with the benign cowpox produced cross-immunity against the more serious smallpox. This spelt the end of the riskier inoculation and was to lead ultimately to the eradication of smallpox. But because of fear of and resistance to the technique, and the initial absence of systematic campaigns immunizing the entire population victory over smallpox came slowly. As late as the 1870s there were still pesthouses, and people disfigured by smallpox remained a common sight in all Sussex towns and villages (see **Typhoid**).

# SNAILS, Syrup of

I'm not sure if the French penchant for escargots renders them less prone to bronchial and pulmonary troubles, but a broth, liquor or syrup made from snails used to be a traditional Sussex cure for colds, catarrh, coughs, bronchitis, 'flu, whooping cough, and even consumption (TB). The earliest example I have come across is this recipe copied into Edward Austin of Burwash's *Book of Receipts*:

> 'Of quick [live] snails, newly taken out of their shelly cottages; of elderberries dried in the oven, and pulverized; and of common salt, of each as much as you will; put it in the straining Bagg, called *Hippocrates* sleave, making one row upon another, so off on as you please; so that the first be of the snails, the next of the salt, and the last of the berries, continuing so till the bagg be full; hang it up in a Cellar and gather diligently the glutinous liquor that distils out of it little by little.'

Two centuries later broths and sirrups of snails were still widely used in the treatment of coughs, whooping cough and consumption, eg this in the Revd Gordon's *History and Natural History of Harting*, 1877:

> 'If, however, the snail should be so fortunate as to escape a fatal accident before it has arrived at maturity, each individual deposits upwards of a hundred eggs, and if its value in the French Pharmacopeia is really as great as it is made out to be, many a sufferer from pulmonary disease has good reason to rejoice at its prolific nature. It is from this species that the invaluable helicine is obtained, but it can scarcely, it seems, be deemed a recent discovery. Without having the faintest suspicion that her specific was destined to be introduced to the medical profession under a scientific name, MATERFAMILIAS, of Harting, has been in the habit of administering it for generations past with the happiest results, in cases of whooping cough

148

and consumption. The formula according to which she prepares it no doubt differs materially from that of the eminent physicians under the sanction of whose name it has taken so high a rank in the MATERIA MEDICA. She simply strings a dozen or so of live snails together, by passing a needle and stout thread through the shell and body of each, these are next suspended festoon-like over a dish or pan containing a layer of coarse brown sugar, in which the mucilaginous fluid exuding from the snails is allowed to drip. The resulting compound is a Syrup of Snails, of which she prescribes two spoonfuls *pro dos*: twice a day. We cannot but suspect that in this custom science has taken a leaf from her.'

'D.M.' of Polegate, in a letter to the *Sussex County Magazine* in 1935 about cures used in rural Sussex during her childhood, noted.

'For those suffering from colds, SNAILS soaked in sugar made the best antidote, and WOODLICE soaked in wine were the asty remedy for dropsy. For gunshot wounds 'boiled WHELPS and EARTHWORMS were used!'

In another letter to the SCM in 1935, Amy Sawyer of Ditchling wrote 'a friend had a bad cough which no doctor's medicine would cure. An old lady said she could cure it if he'd take her stuff. Best results: cough gone. Asked out of curiosity what the potion was made of. On getting the answer "mostly snails", my friend left hurriedly.'

A piece on 'Personalities of Remote Sussex – Mrs Paddick' in the SCM in 1932 has the following dialogue:

' "Your cough seems much better," I ventured. "Yes, and I did cure that myself with snails. I caught a lot down in my rockwork and did pound them up in a basin and take a spoonful at a time, and the cough he was gone in less than a week".

'I endeavoured to conceal the horror I felt and murmured something suitable.

149

"Now your father he's very bronchial. If he would take snails now it would do him a world of good, and if you would rub them into that nasty scratch now it would stop it turning sceptical".'

In 16th to 20th century Sussex the swallowing of live frogs or administering of syrups made by impaling them over a bowl of sugar, and their application, again live, to wounds, were also popular cures for bronchial and pulmonary complaints, and for cuts and wounds (see **Frogs**); and clearly there are shared features linking the frog and snail cures.

Snails and frogs are both covered in mucus and here are being used to cure bronchial/pulmonary complaints characterized by the production of abnormal amounts or kinds of mucus. Both breathe through their skins, which function as, and have the appearance of, pulmonary surfaces, and here they are being used to treat complaints of the pulmonary system. All of this must be more than coincidence.

What we have here are more examples of the age-old practice of using like to cure like. The reasons for doing so were many, various, and usually below the level of conscious explanation, but crudely classifiable into: the homeopathic principle that like has an affinity of like, is drawn to like, hence that like can be used to draw out like (here using the mucus-covered snail or frog to draw to itself and thus draw out infected mucus and with it the infection, or to attract a disease of mucus to itself); the very similar scapegoat principle (that pulmonary snails and frogs are suitably attractive scapegoats for the transference of pulmonary disease); and the way of thinking which lay behind the Doctrine of Signatures (the pulmonary character of snails and frogs signs that they had been placed on Earth as, that part of their raison d'etre was to be, cures for pulmonary disease). For any or all of these reasons, it *felt right* to use pulmonary snails and frogs to treat pulmonary disease.

But it's possible to go a layer deeper than this. Because

snails and frogs are pulmonary in character, and breathe through their skins, they need effective defences against the viruses, bacteria and fungi which pullulate all around them in air, water, and soil. And research confirms that snails and frogs do indeed secrete, are obliged to secrete, powerful microbicides. The chemical defences of snails don't have a collective name, those of frogs are known as maganins, from a Hebrew word for shield.

Though none of these chemicals, unfortunately, has much effect on cold or 'flu viruses, they are lethal to a wide range of bacteria and fungi responsible for bronchial/pulmonary conditions, notably the *Haemophilus* pertussis bacillus responsible for whooping cough, and the *Myobacterium* tuberculosis bacillus. It is therefore possible that preparations made from snails or frogs were useful against some of the maladies for which they were prescribed.

It seems, then, that our ancestors started taking preparations made from snails or frogs for reasons which we would regard as spurious – the same reasons which led them to swallow shivery, shiver-inducing spiders to draw out their shivery agues – only to find, as much by luck as judgement, a family of remedies some of which really did work.

The skin chemicals of snails and frogs are also lethal to many of the bacteria and fungi which cause the septicaemia of cuts and wounds whence the use of frogs as living bandages (see **Frogs**) and of pounded snails (as in the remedies of Mrs Paddick, quoted above) as a cure for wounds.


# SWALLOWS, SWALLOW WATER AND OWL BROTH

Swallows have been used medicinally in places as far removed in time and space as Ancient China, Ancient Greece, and 18th century Sussex. Lei Hiao (AD 420-477) gives the following recipe:

'To use dragon's bone, first boil some aromatic herbs. Wash the bone twice in hot water, then reduce it to powder and place it in tiny bags of thin material. Take two young swallows and, after removing their entrails, stuff the bags into the swallows and hang them over a spring. After one night take the bags out of the swallows, remove the powder and mix it with a preparation for strengthening the kidneys. The effect of such a medicine on disorders of the mind is as if it were divine.'

Cyranides recommended swallowing swallows for epilepsy (the fact that the Chinese and Classical use of swallows were for the same class of ailments suggests that we should be looking for an obvious underlying logic to their use); and Willoughby, in his *Ornithology*, 1678, tells how to cure this disorder with a concoction made from 100 swallows, 1 oz castor oil, and white wine. Similar prescriptions appear in *Mistress Jane Hussey's Still-Room Book* (1692), and in Edward Austin's *Book of Receipts* (Burwash, East Sussex, 1701):

'How to make swallow water. Take 40 or 50 swallows when they are ready to fly, bruise them to pieces in a mortar, feathers and all together, you should put them alive into the mortar. Add to them 1 oz of castorum in powder, put all these in a still with white wine vinegar. Distill it as any other water. You may give 2 or 3 spoonfulls at a time. [This concoction] is very good for the passion of the heart, for the passion of the mother, for the falling sickness [epilepsy], for sudden sounding fitts, for the dead palsie, for apoplexies, lethargies and every other distemper and madness of the head. It comforteth the brain.'

At first reading, these recipes may seem to be of no more than curiosity value. After all, stills are not an everyday household item. And catching 100 swallows surely verges on the impossible, like catching cuckoos (see **Cuckoo**).

But, in fact, 16th-18th century inventories and wills show that a very high proportion of better-off households did possess stills for the preparation of liquors and remedies (and people too poor to have stills often prepared similar recipes involving maceration in place of distillation). And, back in those times, just about every farmhouse, cottage and town house had swift, swallow or martin nests under the eaves.

Living part of the year in a village house in Southern France which has half a dozen swallow nests under its eaves, I know how easy it would be to lean out of a window or put a ladder against the wall and catch large numbers of nesting swallows and their nestling/fledgelings within a very short time.

I have also come across one reference to 'swallow oyl', this in a recipe jotted into small farmer Timothy Butt of Tillington's *Account Books*, c1765-1800:

'For a Strain or a Bruise – One ounce of oyl of Turcomtine [turps], one oz of Oyl of Exeter, one ounce of Oyl of Swallows, one of ointment of Mash Mallad [the plant marsh mallow] one ounce of Nurb oyntment. Mealt it all together then anoint the place.'

It's evident to us today that ingesting swallows or swallow water would be no good for epilepsy. Belief in swallows as a remedy for epilepsy and disturbed mental states seems to go back to the notions of classical writers who associated the bird with frenzied, unintelligible speech because of its rapid twittering: witness the myth of Philomela whose tongue was cut out to stop her talking after she had been dishonoured by her sister's husband, and who was later changed by the gods into a swallow (or, in some accounts, nightingale).

Just as it was thought that swallowing or wearing shivery, shiver-inducing spiders or taking preparations made from the shivering trembling aspen might cure the shivering ague, on the basis of using like to cure like, so it may have been thought that swallowing swallows with their disturbed unintelligible twittering might cure disorders characterized

153

by disturbed, frenzied, unintelligible patterns of behaviour and speech. Unless the notion travelled along the trade routes linking the Ancient Mediterranean and China, it would appear that the Chinese and Greeks arrived independently at the same conclusion.

Rural cures involving birds are few compared with those using plants or insects, no doubt because many plants and insects do possess genuine medicinal virtues, whereas birds do not.

One oft-quoted Sussex cure involved giving a broth made from owls to children suffering from whooping cough. It is difficult to know whether this was on the like-curing-like principle of using the whooping, hooting owl to cure the whooping cough; or whether it was felt that because the owl could whoop away without coming to any harm it might somehow confer this immunity on the child suffering from whooping cough.

Easier to understand is the age-old practice of taking preparations made from birds or the eyes of birds – in theory eagle or raven, in practice magpies, jackdaws, or even chickens – to improve eyesight or cure blindness. Eating the eyes of owls or owls' eggs charred and powdered, or applying various parts of the owl to the eyes as an ointment, should give excellent night vision. The principle here is the ancient one of sympathetic magic, of assimilating the qualities of an animal – in the case of a bird its legendary powers of vision; night vision in owls – by assimilating some appropriate part of its body. Owls' eggs eaten before the event were thought to be a good aversion therapy against drunkenness.

# Thrush

According to one of Mrs Latham's informants, thrush, a disease of the mouth and throat in children, could be cured if a 'left twin' blew three times into the child's mouth – a 'left twin' being one of a pair of which the other had died.

Another informant claims that the blowing had to be done by someone who had been born a posthumous child, and must be repeated three days running, the patient fasting all the while.

In both cases the healer's particularity is that he or she has survived the death of someone very closely linked with him or her. Perhaps he or she was presumed to be endowed with a double portion of the breath of life in consequence?

## Toadeaters

No fair in 17th or 18th century Sussex was complete without a toady or toad-eater: a man who swallowed toads for his living.

Toad-eaters, for the most part, were ill-paid hirelings who travelled from village to village, fair to fair and market to market in the retinue of a mountebank or itinerant quack doctor 'swallowing live toads, popularly supposed to be poisonous, in order to make their employers effect seemingly miraculous cures.'

After the toady had swallowed a toad, slumped to the ground or to the boards of the mountebank's stage in a theatrical faint, had a dose of the quack's cure-all forced through his dying lips and come back miraculously from the threshold of death, the triumphant mountebank would make his way through the gaping gawping gullible crowd doing good business selling little vials of his marvellous remedy with its proven powers against poison.

The operation could, it seems, be a lucrative one, for the mountebank if not for his toad-eaters, as witness this entry in the diary of the East Hoathly tradesman Thomas Turner on 9th July 1760:

'In the afternoon my wife walked to Whitesmith to see a mountybank and his toad-eaters perform wonders, who has a stage built there and comes once a week to cuzen a parcel of poor deluded creatures out of their money by selling his packets, which are to cure people of more distempers than they had in their lives for 1s each, by which means he takes sometimes £8 or £9 of a day.'

While, as this and most other references to toad-eating suggest, toadies were typically jack-puddings – part of the entourage of buffoons or dependents attending on a mountebank – toad-eating might also be practised by quacks, charlatans or saltimbanques to impress or entertain a crowd and/or demonstrate their immunity to poison. Here, for example, in a letter dated June 1768, is Gilbert White of Selborne (*Natural History*, 1789, and see also the entry from John Rous's diary later):

'And I well remember the time, but was not an eye witness to the fact (though numbers of persons were), when a quack of this village ate a toad to make the country people stare; afterwards he drank oil.'

Mountebanks were often popular figures in the Merry England of ballad singers, bear wards, bonesetters, buffoons, charlatans, clowns comedians, conjurors, geomancers, hocus pocus men, jugglers, mandrake men, merry andrews, puppet masters, rope dancers, saltimbanques, tooth-drawers, and tumblers. But their servile dependents the toadies with their nauseating trade of swallowing live toads were the lowest of the low:

'Be the most scorn'd Jack-Pudding in all the pack,
And turn Toad-Eater to some foreign quack'
(Thomas Brown: *Satires on Quackery*, 1704).

Before the 18th century was halfway through, toady and toad-eater had taken on their secondary meaning 'fawning flatterer, sycophant, creep':
'David begged an Explanation of what she meant by a Toad-Eater,' writes Sarah Fielding (sister of Henry), in

156

*The Adventures of David Simple in Search of a Faithful Friend* (1744), 'and Cynthia replied "it is a Metaphor taken from a Mountebank's Boy's eating Toads, in order to show his Master's skill in expelling Poison. It is built on a Supposition that People who are in a State of Dependence, are forced to do the most nauseous things that can be thought on to please their Patrons".'

Here are some further examples of 18th century usage: 'I have got Charles into such order that he toad-eats me beyond conception' (Lady Sarah Lennox, *Life and Letters*, 1766); 'the delight of being toad-eated by all India from Cabul to Assam' *The Life of the Right Hon. William Pitt, with Extracts from his Unpublished Correspondence and Manuscript Papers* (Vol. III, p191) by Philip Henry, 5th Earl Stanhope (1861-2); 'The Beauclercks, Lord Westmorland, and a Mr Jones his tutor or toad-eater were of our party' (Georgiana, Duchess of Devonshire, 26 July 1776).

Though there are many passing references to toad-eaters in 17th and 18th century sources, there is little that provides insight into some of the things one would most like to know about toad-eating; notably a problem that has exercised toxicologists with a knowledge of toad venoms – whether toadies really did swallow toads?

No 17th or 18th century source explicity raises the possibility that toadies may not have swallowed toads (though a doubt on this point may be hinted at in the Walter Gale of Mayfield quote below) – that it might all be sleight of hand deceiving the eye – and several of the accounts by observers who came close to toadies suggest that they really did swallow their toads. Here, for example, is the Suffolk diarist John Rous in 1629:

'I inquired of him if William Utting the toade-eater did not once keepe at Laxfield; he tould me yes, and said he had seene him close by eate a toade.'

And here is an extract from the *Journal* of Mayfield schoolmaster Walter Gale in 1758:

'Master Eastwood, who had been at Frantfield Fair, came to the school: he invited me to the Oak, and treated me with a mugg of fivepenny. Confirm'd he had stood close and seen the mountybanks Jack Pudding swallow his toad, but his seeming dying and wonderful resurrection to health a trick to gull the poor and credulous.'

If one accepts, as these accounts suggest, that toadies did swallow toads, this raises intriguing problems – because toads really are very poisonous.

The warty skin of the common toad is a marvellous miniaturized munitions factory producing a battery of irritants, hallucinogens (eg bufotenin, one of the active ingredients of the witch's mind-altering potions), and heart-stopping cardiac glycosides up to 50 times more potent than digitalis (bufadienolides such as bufotalin). When the toad is attacked by a rat, a fox, or a dog, say, muscles around the warts contract, squeezing out acrid milky venom. The dog, if it isn't deterred by the odour of venom, seizes the toad and immediately drops it, heart pounding, foaming at the mouth, and whimpering with anguish and, if it has any sense, learns the lesson it was intended to learn: THIS ANIMAL IS TABOO! There are many records of dogs dying as a result of biting or attempting to swallow toads.

As long ago as Roman times, women were using toads to poison their husbands. The method of extracting the venom was to throw live toads into a pan of boiling water. The venom came to the top and could be skimmed off. By the 16th century Italian poisoners had perfected a method of incorporating toad venom into salt that could be sprinkled on to a victim's food without detection.

Witches' potions were made by sweltering toads with fat in a stewpot. The ointment this yielded was worked into sensitive areas of the skin, allowing slow absorption of the mind-altering hallucinogens dopamine, serotonin and bufotenin. With the help of a little autosuggestion the witch who worked sweltered toad venom into her skin really did find herself shape-shifting into a familiar or flying through the night sky on her broomstick. The witch's potions were

158

never broths to be taken internally, because the witch who drank a broth made from toads would have risked dropping dead.

This knowledge about the toxicology of toad venoms provokes a couple of questions about the practical aspects of toad-eating.

First, how were toadies able to swallow toads when their poisons are there precisely to prevent swallowing – by any predator, whether a rat, a dog, or a toad-eater and, from the evidence of biology and natural history are very effective at preventing swallowing? Victorian scientists who bit on and tried to swallow toads in the interests of science experienced immediate unbearable symptoms (shooting pains in the head, numbness of lips and tongue, uncontrollable flow of saliva, delirium, nausea, juddering heart and chest pains) and concluded that it would have been physically impossible for toadies to swallow toads.

The answer, I suspect, is that the toad with its equable temperament only sweats poison when it is desperately frightened, when approached or bitten by something which is obviously a predator. Toads seldom sweat poison when handled by gardeners. The first art of toad-eating must have consisted in pampering the toad, bringing it gently to the lips, and then swallowing it down all of a sudden before it could become alarmed and sweat poison.

Second, having swallowed his toad, why didn't the toady drop down dead from heart failure? Well, biochemists – interested in the applications of bufadienolides in treating heart disease (the ancient Chinese used an extract of toad venom known as *Ch'an su* to treat heart disease, as we use digitalis) – have worked out the concentrations of bufadienolides in toad venom, the doses of orally administered bufadienolides which can be safely given to patients, and the doses above which lethal effects become likely. Their results suggest that a toady who swallowed a single small toad after a good meal was running little risk (at worst he might end up with a terrible headache). A toady who swallowed a large toad or several small toads in a short space of time risked an unpleasant demise.

Despite their formidable venoms, toads have many enemies. Grass snakes, specialist predators on amphibians, are partially immune to the skin poisons deployed by European newts, frogs and toads. Though they seem to prefer the more palatable common frog or smooth and palmate newts, rejecting great crested newts and toads during times of plenty, there are many records of grass snakes preying on toads, particularly when other prey is unavailable.

Loveridge has described how he watched a brown rat tear the skin off a live toad to get at the flesh underneath, and there are other accounts of hedgehogs, weasels, stoats, badgers and foxes disembowelling toads with their claws. Similarly, rooks, crows, jackdaws, magpies, buzzards, herons and gulls disembowel toads with their beaks, eating the toad from the inside out before discarding the skin. As there are also records of all these animals rejecting toads, it would appear that this is a copied, or intelligent and not instinctive, behaviour.

# TREES

It used to be a common belief that many conditions could be cured by bringing the sufferer into contact with the powerful life force or mana represented by trees – the more so if the tree was one which had held a place in ancient religions, like the oak or the ash, or a role in Christian symbolism, like the thorn – in order to effect a transfer of that life force. One drastic example was recorded by the Revd Henry Hoper, Rector of Portslade from 1815 to 1889, in a note discovered and published by his grand-daughter Miss E.G. Hoper:

'Singular supersition exists at Portslade near Brighton and has been entertained within the memory of man, namely, that a dying person can be recovered if thrice carried round, and then banged against, a thorn of great antiquity,

160

which stands on the downs ever ready to dispense its magical power to all believers. A few years ago a medical attendant gave up all hopes for his patient. The Goodies of the village obtained the Doctor's and the sick man's consent to restore him to health, and having carried him round the tree, bumped the dying man, and had the mortification of carrying him away a corpse, much to their astonishment at the ill success of their specific.'

Some years later Mrs Latham noted a widespread belief that the maple tree confers its life on any sick or dying child passed between its branches. There was one in West Grinstead Park in her time, and she observed that much rage and distress was caused by a rumour that it was to be cut down. She also refers to the belief that one could cure oneself of fits (or, some said, of boils) by crawling three times through the arch formed by a branch which had curled over and re-rooted itself at the tip.

The best documented procedure of this type was the one used to cure a child of a hernia by passing it through a cleft made with an axe in an ash sapling, the cleft then being bound up and allowed to grow together again. The tree chosen for this ritual, the ash, was regarded as being powerful against snakes, shrews, and similar manifestations of evil. Here is Mrs Latham's account.

'A child so afflicted must be passed 9 times in succession on 9 successive days at sunrise through a cleft in a sapling ash tree, which has been so far given up by the owner of it to the parents of the child that there is an understanding that it should not be cut down during the life of the child that is to be passed through it. The sapling must be sound at heart, and the cleft must be made with an axe. The child being carried to the tree must be attended by 9 persons, each of whom must pass it through the cleft from west to east. On the 9th morning the solemn ceremony is concluded by binding the tree tightly with a cord, and it is supposed that as the cleft closes the health

161

of the child will improve. In the neighbourhood of Petworth some cleft ashes may be seen, through which children have very recently been passed. I may add that only a few weeks since, a person who had lately purchased an ash tree standing in this parish [Fittleworth], intending to cut it down, was told by the father of a child who had some time before been passed through it, that the infirmity would be sure to return upon his son if it were felled. Whereupon the good man said, he knew such would be the case, and that therefore he would not fell it for the world.'

Similar trees could be found in most rural parishes in Sussex, and until a very late date. Percy Goodman, for example, writing in the *Sussex Archaeological Collections* in the 1920s, commented:

'This superstition obtained until recently in this neighbourhood, and we have more than one tree still to be seen which shows signs of having been treated in this way. We have a tree still standing within a few yards of the boundary of this parish, and the man is still living on the farm in which the tree is, who passed through this ordeal.'

In this ritual the splitting of the tree imitates the rupture from which the child is suffering, and hence the subsequent healing of the tree is supposed to promote the child's; magic numbers are used, and a persistent magical connection is set up between the child's destiny and that of the tree (see also **Ague, Shrew Ash, Warts**).

## TYPHOID, CHOLERA

The populations of most Sussex towns increased steeply during the 18th and 19th centuries. This brought with it an increase in the incidence of diseases such as smallpox, associated with contagion; and of typhoid and cholera, linked with contaminated water, poor sanitation, and inadequate waste disposal. Ever-increasing quantities of effluvia from household privies, cess pits and middens, uncontrolled public dumps, abattoirs, butchers' shops and so on seeped into the soil, contaminating the streams, springs and wells from which the population drew its drinking water. Smallpox was always present, and there were major outbreaks of cholera or typhoid which caused many fatalities in Chichester, Lewes, Rye and Worthing. Here is an extract from a portrait of Chichester, entitled *Chichester 60-65 Years Ago*, published by Thomas Parsons in 1934, which gives something of the flavour of life in a Sussex town in the 19th century:

> 'Chichester, 60 or 65 years ago, was a terrible place. Deformed and degenerate persons were numerous. People disfigured by that terrible disease, smallpox, or as it was sometimes called, the white plague, were numerous. On the eastern end of the city, outside the walls, there was a hospital for such patients. This was known as the Pest House. Typhoid fever abounded. It was not uncommon to find two or three cases in one house at the same time. The road outside the house would be covered thick with tar to deaden the sound of passing traffic. The cause of this disease was found in the drinking water of the houses, which was drawn or pumped from wells which were in some cases within 10 feet of an open cess pit . . .
>
> 'The stream of the Lavant ran through the city behind many of the houses. Where the present Market Road now is, it formed an open ditch, beside which was a pathway leading to the fields. These were known as the Hunston Meadows. In the dry season this ditch was the receptacle for refuse and dead cats and dogs.'

Smaller towns suffered outbreaks too. Here is the *West Sussex Gazette* of 7 September 1893:

'We regret to say that Arundel is being visited by an outbreak of typhoid fever, though, as yet, fortunately, of too limited an extent to cause undue alarm. The first cases occurred some three weeks back, in houses in Tarrant Street, and were attributed to the use of water from a well close to Mr Chives' premises, water which has now been declared to be impure, but which has been permitted to be freely used for years. One of the earliest of the cases, that of the young Volunteer Skinner, terminated fatally, and on Tuesday of this week, when the total of cases had risen up to 13, a second case reached a fatal ending. Prompt measures are being taken to isolate the patients, and owing to the generosity of the Duke of Norfolk, the St Phillip's Club has been expeditiously and most adequately fitted up as a hospital, which was opened on Wednesday, under the control of the Town Council.'


## VIPERS AND VIPER-CATCHERS

Snakes – adders for preference, but sometimes grass snakes – were one of the staples of early (Ancient, Medieval, Renaissance to early Georgian) and rural folk medicine. We have only occasional glimpses into their use in 15th-18th century Sussex, but a great deal more information on methods of viper-catching and the preparation and use of viper-based remedies in 19th and early 20th century.

'If I could hear as well as see,/No man would be the death of me' runs an old Sussex rhyme about the adder, recorded in several villages during the 19th century. On the homeopathic principle of using like to cure like, preparations made from the deaf adder were used as remedies for deafness and other ailments of the ears.

In Elizabethan Sussex, vipers boiled in wine were a popular remedy for earache. And as recently as the 1920s-1940s viper venom, viper blood, and viper fat melted down to give an oil, were still employed in many isolated villages to treat deafness, earache, and mastoids.

Here, for example, is a letter from Edmund Austen published in the *Sussex County Magazine* in 1935:

'In reading Miss Robinson's charming recollections of her childhood, I was interested in the reference to her father's payment of sixpence for every adder killed on his land.

'As a boy, I remember that my great uncle, the late Mr Horace Coleman, of Chitcombe, Brede, gave a similar sum for each adder killed on his estate, and in addition three pence for every snake. This resulted in their numbers being greatly diminished – in fact, for many years past, the sight of an adder has been a rare occurrence.

'I wonder whether Mr Robinson made a similar use of the dead adders as did Mr Coleman's gamekeeper – a venerable old gentleman named Fred Furminger. He would extract, during the summer months, the 'fleed' (or inside fat) from selected adders, and suspend them on nails on the front wall of his cottage, which faced south. Underneath would be placed small bottles to catch the drops of oil as the fat was melted by the rays of the sun.

'Those little bottles hanging in a row often aroused the curiosity of visitors. The oil was very precious, being a wonderful specific for deafness. A few drops placed in the ear have been known to cure quite a number of obstinate cases. Folk came from miles around to buy a small quantity from the old gamekeeper. On one occasion, I remember using a few drops myself with satisfactory result.'

Five to seven dead adders were generally required to fill one small bottle with oil.

And here is an even more recent account of the use of snake preparations to cure ailments of the ear, sent to me by Mrs Pat Rodmore of Felpham:

'When a child of 10 to 11 years, I developed mastoids in both ears. I was very sick at the time and our old family doctor gave my mother adders' blood, two drops had to be put on a warmed small silver spoon and then into each ear. I cannot now remember how many days this lasted but I can well remember my mother telling me it was 10/6d a drop! This was in 1927/8 and we were far from affluent. It cured the mastoids and with fingers crossed I have had no further trouble. I can remember the little bottle and the drops were red in colour like blood. I was horrified as I have never been able to like snakes of any kind, but must say my cure for mastoids without the operation has made me feel indebted to the adder.'

By this time adder preparations had long since lost their place in the official *Materia Medica*: Mrs Rodmore's doctor was prescribing an archaic remedy which his predecessors in Stuart or Georgian times might have prescribed, but now in the border zone nearer to apothecary's/traditional rural medicine.

The astounding price of the drops helps explain why, even if faith in traditional rural cures was waning, many people shunned professional doctors for all but the most serious conditions, turning instead to the advice of the local wise woman or to remedies handed down within their community. Even at this late date, adder oil or adder blood could still have been obtained much more reasonably from the equivalent of Mr Coleman's gamekeeper.

The sloughed skin of a snake was also believed to be effective against earache. Here, for example, is the Hampshire and West Sussex botanist John Goodyer, writing in the 17th century:

'The Senecta Anguium (which is the skinne that ye snake casts in ye spring tyme) being sod with wine, is a remedy for ye paine in the ears if it be poured into them, and for ye pain of the teeth when taken by way of collation.'

Preparations made from snakes were used to treat a vast range of conditions, extending far beyond the obvious deafness/earache. To understand why snakes were regarded as a panacea for just about every ailment known to man –

including old age itself – we must go back far beyond the medieval period. The origins of many of the snake remedies recorded in Sussex during the 15th-20th centuries can be traced back to Mesopotamia and Sumer many millenia ago. The earliest medical text known to archaeologists is a Sumerian clay tablet from the 3rd millenium BC including remedies made from snakes and snake skins.

Our far-off ancestors watched with awe – and envy – the snake that could shed its old skin and thereby renew its youth, emerging from its slough larger, stronger, and more brilliantly coloured than before; the snake that could be reborn an infinite number of times and seemed to posses the secret of living forever. They associated the snake with immortality and eternal youth, as in this passage from the 12th century *Revesby Abbey Bestiary*:

'Snakes live for ever, the reason being that, when they have sloughed off their old skins, it is granted to them to cast off their old age and return to youth.'

And they hoped that by taking preparations made from snakes they could assimilate the secret of eternal, or at least long, life – hence the cure-all quality of snake preparations – and glowing healthy skin, whence the traditional use of snake preparations as cosmetics and in the treatment of skin conditions such as leprosy and lupus.

Our old friend John Goodyer had this to say about the virtues of adder flesh and adder salts:

'The flesh of the viper being sod, and eaten, makes the eyes quick-sighted, and it is good also for the griefs of the Nerves, and it doth repress the increasing Strumae . . . some say that in feeding on them lice are bred in such as eate them, but it is a lye. Some about me here say that they who eate them are long-lived.'

And here is his account of how adder salts were prepared in the 17th century:

'The living viper is put into a pot and with it salt and dry figs well beaten with honey. The cover of the pot is close stopt with clay and they are baked in an Oven till the salt be turned to water. And sometimes that it may agree better with ye Stomach there is some Spikenard or a little Malabrathrum mixed with it.'

Because of their association with rejuvenation and glowing skin it was natural that snakes should be used for cosmetic purposes. In his *Historie of Serpentes* (1658), the Revd Edward Topsell writes 'The blood of a serpente is more precious than Balsamum, and if applied to the lips, this will look passing red, and if the face be anointed therewith, it will receive no spot or fleck, but cometh to have an orient or beautiful hue.' Venetia Stanley, one of the most noted beauties of the 17th century, wife of the diplomat-author Sir Kenelm Digby, put the advice into practice by dining every day on capons fed with viper flesh.

Because of its rejuvenating effect on the skin, viper flesh was widely used in the treatment of leprosy, common in Anglo-Saxon and medieval Sussex and on into the 17th and 18th centuries. In his *De Proprietatibus Rerum* (1240), Bartolamaeus Anglicus, English Bartholomew, writes 'to heal leprosy or hide it the best remedy is a red adder with a white belly if the venom is away and the head smitten off. Then the body sodden with leeks should be taken and eaten often.' Dr Meade, in his *Mechanical Art of Poison* (1702), quoted evidence from Galen and Pliny to justify the use of adder flesh in the treatement of goitre and leprosy.

In many Sussex villages as recently as a century ago snakes were still being used to treat goitre. At Withyam, according to Lilian Candlin, it was the practice to draw a live snake three times across the swelling. The snake was then left to crawl around for a time. This was repeated three times so that the snake was drawn across the neck nine times: nine being a powerful magic number encountered in several other entries. It was then put into a tightly sealed bottle and buried in the ground. As the snake rotted, the swelling on the neck would gradually die down (see **Slug**).

A similar remedy was used in a nearby village. Here a dead snake was wrapped in a silk scarf after it had been skinned, and the sufferer had to wear it constantly around his or her neck until the swelling subsided.

For a more gruesome cure for goitre see **Gibbet**.

In Elizabethan Sussex people tied snake sloughs around their backs to guard against rheumatism and wore snake skin belts against backache. Three centuries later, in 1877, the Revd D.A. Gordon, in his *History and Natural History of Harting*, noted 'we have often found the slough between the stems of dead ferns and other rigid plants, but until recently we were quite ignorant of its value. We now know that many persons suffering from headache have used it as a bandage across the forehead for the purpose of "charming away" the pain'. Just before the First World War, a little old man still toured the villages between Midhurst and Selborne selling snake sloughs which, tied across the temples, were said to be an excellent cure for headaches.

Until the middle of the 18th century doctors throughout Sussex prescribed snake preparations for a vast range of ills, major or minor, country people used much the same preparations; and every apothecary sold viper venom, viper blood, viper oil, viper fat, viper ointment (a mixture of viper oil and lard used, appropriately, for adder bites; and for rheumatism and as a cure for warts), and sloughs. The demand for vipers was so great that the local supply couldn't keep up and they had to be imported from Italy. In the 1660s viper oil fetched £11 an oz at an apothecary in Chichester, this at a time when the average agricultural wage was £4-£8 a year. We can deduce that the trade of local viper catcher, whether professional or part-time, must have been a lucrative one – much more lucrative than farm labour – and that pressure on viper populations must have been extreme.

By the 1740s, faith in snake preparations among the medical fraternity was waning. In 1745, the now venerable

Dr Meade complained that physicians were becoming too sparing in their prescription of viper broth. They prescribed a few grams of dried viper, when the patient really needed frequent platefuls of steaming viper broth, or viper *à l'ancienne*, boiled whole and eaten like fish.

By 1800 few doctors were prescribing snake preparations and the heyday of the professional viper catchers was nearing its end. But the demand for viper products from apothecaries (who operated in a twilight zone between official and popular medicine) and the rural population remained high, and throughout the 19th and into the 20th century viper-catching remained a lucrative side-line for farm labourers, gamekeepers, and small boys – particularly as agricultural wages were so low and much of the rural population lived in a desperate poverty reflected in violent popular uprisings such as the 'Captain Swing' riots.

A couple of accounts of the methods used to catch adders have come down to us. First, here is a letter from Mr Maurice Burns of Slindon:

'George was born in 1804 and was employed as a young man on the Parham Park Estate. In 1892 he told his grandson (my father Joseph Burns, then aged 11) that when he was a little boy living in W. Chiltington he used to catch adders for old Dame Jackson who was said to be a witch.

'She said she could cure not only earache, toothache and bellyache but also rheumatism if you paid her enough and bought enough adders' fat and rubbed it in where it hurt.

'George used to catch adders for her with little bits of red flannel tied on to long pieces of string, which he pulled along over dried leaves where they lay on the ground in woods.

'The adders would dart out and bite the flannel which got caught on their little teeth which point inwards down their throats.

'When he felt a tug on the string, he caught hold of the adder and pulled the flannel out of its throat, with the two teeth and little bags of poison still caught in the flannel.

This made it harmless, and Dame Jackson used to give him a penny for every adder he brought her. With the money he bought ducks' eggs at two for a penny.'

And here is a second account from *Round About Sussex Downs* by Frederick Wood, 1935:

'Poynings Woods and some rough ground near is a very favourite place with the reptiles. Years ago an old man used to collect them here with a forked stick. He then extracted the oil, which was used by the old folk as a cure for deafness, and I believe it is a very good remedy.'

In the 1890s, a local viper catcher regularly sold viper fat to an apothecary in Uckfield for a guinea an ounce. In real terms the price of vipers and viper fat had fallen compared with the 16th century, but viper-catching was still a lucrative part-time trade.

# WALNUTS

Such a nice tree, you say: dark pinnate leaves, rather attractive grey-and-green striped bark, the whole appearance feathery, rather like one of those generalised trees in 18th century watercolours. Why, everyone asks, weren't more walnut trees planted? And fresh green walnuts are so good, the timber valuable and always in demand...But, ah, there were hidden dangers.

In olden time Sussex it was not thought safe to sit beneath a walnut tree – not just because the nuts might fall on your head, but because the tree's effluvium was believed to derange the mind. Sleeping under walnut trees was even more strongly discouraged, leading to madness or death, as in this cryptic Sussex saying recorded by Parish in the 19th century:

'He that would eat the fruit must climb the tree.
He that would eat the kernel must crack the nut.
He that sleepeth under a walnut doth get fitts in
   the head.'

As late as the 19th century walnuts were believed to exert
so baleful an influence that they were never planted near
houses (or strawberry beds or other valuable plants); so if
there's one next to your front door it probably isn't very old,
at least by the standards of this extremely long-lived tree. In
the past they were planted a good distance away, often in the
orchard's shelter belt (but not too close to the fruit trees).
However, they played an important role in the household
economy and medicine chest.

The walnut *Juglans regia* is not native to Britain, but seems
to have been brought by the Romans (they'd got it from the
Greeks who found it growing in Persia, though it is native a
lot further east). Thereafter, it all but disappeared from Britain
– though its name walnut from *wealh nut* or foreign nut is of
Anglo-Saxon origin – and was not widely grown again until
the 16th century, when Leonard Mascal the Plumpton
agriculturist and Thomas Tusser the East Hoathly agriculturist
reintroduced it to Sussex and lauded its many virtues, while
also warning against its malevolent influence.

Fresh nuts, much better than the tired ones we are
subjected to at Christmas, were eaten at the beginning of
meals (which sounds fun), but they were also used as a
vermifuge (which doesn't). Indeed walnuts were originally
pickled so that parasite worms could be expelled throughout
the year. They were also a handy counter-poison.

Less dramatically, they served to suppress onion-scented
belches, and by 1714 were also being used as a sharp sauce
for mackerel and cold meats.

Following the Doctrine of Signatures (the form or markings
of a plant revealing its medicinal qualities) nuts were hung
around the neck to cure 'falling fits' (epilepsy) and other
mental disorders (because the nut, once extracted from the
shell, has a remarkable resemblance to the human brain). The
connection with madness may (or may not) explain why

172

preparations made from walnuts were used to 'know the bite of a madde [ie rabid] dogge (see **Dog**).

18th century greenfly were sprayed with solutions made from walnut leaves and bark (and sometimes henbane and wormwood too), a practice that continued until pyrethrum came into general use. A similar concoction was used to kill worms in the lawn.

This testimony that walnut leaves and bark contain chemicals lethal to other life forms brings us back to the idea that walnut trees exert a baleful influence. The notion that sitting or sleeping under walnut trees might be harmful to health or sanity, or even fatal, wasn't just superstitious nonsense.

As early as the Roman period, Pliny, in his *Naturalis Historia*, noted that bees in hives set under walnuts were stunted and sickly and produced very little honey. He pointed out, too, that walnuts apparently exercise a baleful influence over other plants growing in their vicinity. Modern research has confirmed that the insect and soil fauna under walnuts is atypical and impoverished; and that many plants either die or grow up sickly and stunted if planted within the 'death zone' or zone of influence of a walnut.

This isn't simply because of shading and/or food competition. Many soil insects die if they are placed in earth taken from near walnut trees, and many plants grow sickly and stunted or die if they are grown in such soil.

The walnut tree manufactures and stores in its leaves and bark the precursor form of a chemical called juglone – an 'allelochemical' – which is converted into active juglone by rain and washed down on to the soil. This chemical inhibits seed germination and the growth of other plants. That is, the walnut uses its deadly allelochemical to wage biochemical warfare on the rest of the plant kingdom. Many plants are susceptible to juglone; others, notably some grasses and many brambles and currants, have evolved resistance.

Juglone is lethal to animals too, killing or stunting the growth of insects or other small creatures unfortunate enough to enter the walnut's death zone.

The effect also extends to humans. In the Middle Ages and

173

Renaissance, concoctions of macerated walnut leaves and bark were used to turn children into dwarfs, for sale to courts and travelling fairs and shows. Some idea of the prices being paid for dwarfs, of the profits to be made from 'dwarfing' unwanted or stolen children, can be had from this news item in the *Sussex Weekly Advertiser*, 16 January 1769:

> 'At Rogate, in Sussex, near Petersfield, lives John Ball, who has a son now nineteen years of age, and but forty inches high; he has been offered £100 for him, to shew at fairs which, though in indigent circumstances, so great is his paternal affection for the child, he refused.'

This was at a time when the annual wage for a labourer was no more than £4-£8 per annum.

And here's a quote from the diary of Mr John Baker of Horsham on 18 July 1776, which speaks volumes and doesn't need any commentary:

> 'Horsham Fair. Called in at Mrs Tredcroft, came on Mr Blunt and Uxor, Mr Edward T and two sisters. Ladies had been to see a Monmouthshire girl of 16 not above 33¼ inches high. Her mother shewed her. Said she was 16 a few days ago; well proportioned but face disgustful, large eyes, pale, looks like an abortion, dressed in red riding habit and laced hat.'

As juglone isn't volatile, so doesn't form a miasma and can only be activated by rain, I can't see that there could be any danger sitting or sleeping under walnut trees. But the traditional belief that it might be dangerous so to do was a rational extrapolation from the accurate observation that walnuts undoubtedly do exert a malevolent influence over other animals and plants in their death zone (the French talk of *l'ombre maléfique du noyer*).

174

# Warts and Wartwort

In the entry on **Frogs**, I wrote about maganins: chemicals produced in the skin glands of frogs and toads and secreted on to the surface of the skin at all times, but especially following stress or injury, as a defence against bacterial or fungal infection. I pointed out that these chemicals are lethal to the tuberculosis bacillus, thus the old Sussex custom of swallowing live frogs as a cure for consumption; and lethal to the bacteria responsible for sepsis, therefore the custom of strapping on frogs or toads as living bandages for bad cuts.

But not all traditional cures embody such immemorial wisdom. Witness, for example, the superficially similar practice of applying toads cut in half to warts: popular in Sussex until recent times, and recorded over the centuries from just about everywhere in Europe.

It is easy to understand why country people down the ages have experimented with toads as a cure for warts. First, frogs and toads are an effective cure for cuts and perhaps also for certain forms of skin infection, so it was reasonable to try toads as a possible cure for warts. Second, toads were used because they are seemingly covered with warts (in fact, these are skin glands producing a range of secretions; human warts are benign tumours caused by a papilloma virus). On any of the traditional principles of using like to cure like, or as a scapegoat for transference, or consulting the Doctrine of Signatures it seemed right to use toad warts to cure human warts.

But experiments have shown that while maganins have a powerful bacteriocidal and fungicidal action, they and other components of the frog's or toad's skin secretion have no anti-viral properties, no effect on the virus responsible for warts, no effect on the fate of warts in situ or in tissue culture.

So while it's easy to see why country people experimented with toads for warts, it's less easy to understand why generations of country people persisted in applying toads to their warts when toads are, in reality, quite ineffectual as a cure.

The explanation is straightforward. Warts come and go in

mysterious ways, making it impossible for an ordinary person to know (without investigations involving many patients and complex statistics) whether the disappearance of a wart is the result of a particular treatment or no more than a spontaneous regression

'B' applies a toad to his wart and, lo and behold!, a few weeks later the wart disappears, proving to the local community that toads are a cure for warts. 'C' later tries the same cure – to no avail. As toads are known to be effective against warts, it follows that he has omitted some essential ancillary condition: perhaps the cure only works if the toad is collected at a particular phase of the moon. Thus the number of wart cures tends to increase over time (as more cures are tried and appear to work, earning a place in the corpus of rural medicine) and so does their complexity (as cures which worked in the past mysteriously fail, necessitating the addition of supplementary charms and conditions).

Moles' blood, water collected from hollows in poplar trees at midnight, cobwebs, the white cushiony lining of broad bean pods, adder ointment, woad leaves and juice, boiled teasel roots, cantharidin from blister beetles; all were popular Sussex cures. Casting spells or hexing were equally recommended for the credulous. It was claimed to be especially efficacious to rub the warts with steak, all the better if it was stolen first and buried in secret afterwards; and for the brave, I was told during my Goring-by-Sea childhood, an infallible method is to stick a pin into the centre of the wart and then heat the head of the pin until it is red hot (but sterilize the pin first!).

Looking down my list of some 40 Sussex wart cures, it is obvious that in addition to the like curing like toad principle, most of the cures can be classified into two main groups.

The first, rationally enough, involved the use of plants or animals with corrosive sap or secretions to 'eat away' the warts.

Throughout Sussex, buttercups used to be known as 'wart flowers' on this account as were several other plants such as the sun spurge (*Euphorbia heliscopia*) which was known as

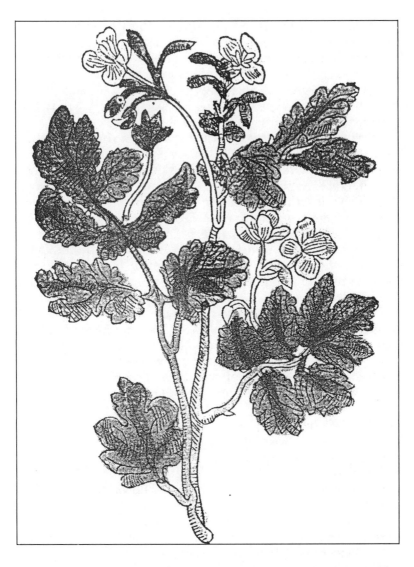

*The greater celandine, a member of the Poppy family and not to be confused with the lesser celandine, a member of the Buttercup family.*

'wartwort' as early as the 16th and into the 19th century, and the petty spurge *E.peplus*, similarly known as wart grass and wart weed. Dandelion sap was used to eat warts, as were the corrosive saps of the red campion, scarlet pimpernel, yellow toadflax, and greater celandine, the latter in Sussex dialect being kill-wart, swallow-wart, wartflower, wartweed (Warzenkraut in German) and yellow spit.

Break a stem of greater celandine and a drop of orange latex oozes out, a drop of that 'yellow spit' which was applied to warts. It is acrid and makes the skin go red, but it is not an effective remedy. Indeed, none of these 'corrosive' treatments is effective, rather the contrary, because they cause damage around the wart, facilitating the spread of the wart virus which can only infect damaged skin.

Elder was another old specific: 'Wartes – wash them with the juice of the berries when the berries be black and doe so every night and so binde them to in the nights' (W. Langham, *The Garden of Health*, 1633). Elder flowers were also used in an ointment. Warts could also be washed in water collected from the teasel or black poplar, while a poultice of onions was believed to draw the warts and break them, like boils. A 17th century remedy mentioned by Turner involved an application of the ashes of willow bark soaked in vinegar, while ashes of cabbage were considered 'very caustick... The juyce cures warts' (J. Floyer *The Touch-stone of Medicines*, 1687). The common mullein was also employed: 'the Juyce of the leaves and flowers being laid upon rough Warts; as also the Pouder of the dryed Roots rubbed on doth easily take them away; but doth no good to smooth Warts'. A poultice of crushed woodbine or honeysuckle laid on the warts was believed to draw and heal them.

A second category of more magical cures for warts took several forms, namely: burial, wedging, nailing, and throwing away. These were invariably combined with the practice of rubbing the warts with sap or counting them.

Burial took the form of rubbing the warts with pieces of plant material which were then placed in a hole dug for this purpose. As the plant decayed so it was believed did the warts; their affinity with the plant lying in the fact that they had been touched by it. Around Crowborough, for example, warts were rubbed nine times with a potato cut into two pieces. The halves were re-united and buried. Near Harting the warts were opened to the quick or till they bled, and then rubbed with the cut surface of a sour apple. The apple was then buried.

A bean shell rubbed on the warts was another remedy; this was secretly buried under an ash tree to the following rhyme:

> 'As this bean shell rots away
> So my wart shall soon decay'

Warts could also be rubbed with a green stick of elder which was then buried, or three drops of blood from the wart were placed on a leaf and this was buried. Another form of the burial practice involved the interment of the same number of seeds or fruits as the person had warts; one common remedy was to touch each wart with a green pea, then bury each pea separately. A variant was to take as many buds from an alder bush as there were warts and bury these.

A related form can be described as wedging, in which the bark of a tree or the wood was opened or slit, and the infection was placed within. The opening was then either closed by pressing the slit back together or otherwise wedging or binding it. Near Lewes the practice was for a person afflicted with warts to go to an ash tree and cut his or her initials in the bark. Then the exact number of warts had to be counted, and as many notches as warts made in the bark, in addition to the letters. As the bark grew over the cuts, the warts would go.

The final form is that of 'nailing', in the sense of driving the infection deep into a tree or other host. Again oaks or ash were favoured, trees considered to have protective qualities. In most cases a pin or nail was the immediate agent. This was used either to probe the infected area and thus anointed with blood, matter or tissue; or laid on the wart; or used to make words or the sign of the cross over the wart before being driven deep into a tree or beam. For example, Mrs Latham

179

tells us that in West Sussex the cure was to prick the warts with pins, then stick the pins into an ash tree; as they became embedded in the growing bark, the warts would gradually disappear. A variant was to stick a pin in an ash tree up to the head and say, in allusion to the belief that one person could 'buy' another's warts

> 'Ashy tree, ashy tree,
> Pray buy these warts off me.'

See also **Cunning Folk: Janet Steer, Slug.**


# WHOOPING COUGH

Whooping cough, it was said, could be cured by any remedy whatever which happened to be recommended by a man riding a piebald horse. Mrs Latham knew a man who had such a horse, and who was constantly being asked to suggest remedies; he would answer quite arbitrarily, and his advice was always taken. Another cure for the same ailment recorded by Haskins in 1931 was to feed the sufferer on bread and butter given by a family where the head of the household was called John and the wife Joan.

For other remedies for this formerly common and life-threatening ailment see **Cow, Horse, Sheep; Elecampane; Frog, Cunning Folk: Grandmother Huggett's Cures; Mice, Snails; Swallow.**


# WORMWOOD, WORMWORT AND WORMSEED

Where general hygiene is poor intestinal parasites abound, especially in the young. Worms (threadworms, roundworms, tapeworms) are a major problem in the developing world today. They were an equally unpleasant commonplace of everyday life in 16th-18th century Sussex, particularly in ports and towns such as Seaford, Rye, Lewes and Chichester, with their overcrowding, poor sanitation, and poverty; but many people in country areas suffered from worms too. Dr Meade, in 1742, describes worming a child in a village near Rye of 47 worms, including two *Tenia* six and eight feet long. And in Walter Gale of Mayfield's *Diary* one finds the following entry, dated Monday 5th February 1751:

'Being very wet in going to town, I went into Peerlesses to dry up, and spent 2d. Here was Satan, who affirmed that his father voided a worm out of his mouth upwards of 5 ells long. He said he could produce a woman in the town who would vouch for the truth of his assertion.'

Men of the pre-industrial period lived in a verminous universe unimaginable today, inhabited by the 'foul and verminous colony', nearly impossible to eradicate, entrenched in their 'sanctuaries', clinging to the narrow cavities of the intestine, masters of the entire territory between throat and sphincter: 'burying into the intestinal walls with fury, they sometimes eat into them, or at least violently distend them, which causes pain, and also from just their wriggling and harshly stiffening up are born the most pernicious symptoms and sometimes even death.'

Apart from the sheer life-draining debilitating unpleasantness of being afflicted with worms, they were thought to be the cause of a wide range of diseases: epilepsy, dizziness, drowsiness, delirium, convulsions, headache, loss of consciousness, palpitations, depression, coughs, vomiting, nausea, diarrhoea, hiccups, pain, colic, wasting away, chronic and acute fevers, and innumerable others. Small wonder then that getting rid of worms occupied a place of honour in the corpus of rural medicine (we know a great deal about the subject of worming in the 17th and 18th centuries, but have little information from the 19th century because the Victorian folklorists who collected information on folk cures remained silent about unmentionable subjects such as worms, venereal diseases, and 'women's troubles').

One dangerous and not very effective, but widely practised, way of worming a child was to administer laxatives. Among the gentler laxatives once popular in Sussex were raw carrots, birch juice, or the juice from the bark of a young fir. Among the less gentle were caper spurge, spurge laurel, dog's mercury, hellebores, and black and white bryony, all real purging purges, but with unpleasant, sometimes lethal side effects. The *Sussex Weekly Advertiser* in 1772 reported the case of a child whose untimely death was attributable to a too-violent worming with caper spurge.

Hellebores in particular were widely collected in the countryside and grown by housewives, partly against boils and spots, partly against worms in children, a drastically, dangerously, and poisonously cathartic purge, as Gilbert White of Selborne recognized, by which the local children were quite often killed. 'Where it killed not the patient' it was said, 'it would certainly kill the worm; but the worst of it is, it will often kill both'.

In the 16th century a sporting element was introduced into worming by 'Merry Andrew' Borde of Pevensey – lapsed Carthusian monk, traveller, versifier, agronomist, brothel owner, mountebank, and physician to Henry VIII. In this a string was tied to a piece of fresh pork and the bait was then introduced into the 'intestinum rectum' of the sufferer. After a short time, the meat could be pulled out again, and with luck and skill a number of the ever hungry worms would come with it. The process was repeated with fresh pieces of pork until all the worms had been evacuated.

Laxatives, purgatives, and fishing with bait were of limited effectiveness for getting rid of worms. But early and rural medicine had also discovered the use of plants – male fern; agrimony; walnuts (see); and the aptly-named wormwoods and wormworts – with powerful vermicidal properties.

*Senecio fluviatilis/sarracenicus*, the 'wormwort', is an alien from southern Europe introduced by the Romans and now naturalized in Sussex. In the 16th-18th centuries it was cultivated in gardens as a source of worming drugs, and grown on plots outside villages and small towns for sale to apothecaries or the London market. It is a powerful vermicide, containing in all its parts a battery of alkaloids with anti-helminthic, vermifugal properties.

Plants of the genus *Artemisia* are collectively known as 'wormwoods'. Three species were commonly used as vermicides in Sussex: maritime wormwood *A.maritimum*, probably a native, once common and collected on a commercial scale along the Sussex coast; mugwort, *A. vulgaris*, either a native or introduced in very early times; and absinthe, *A. absinthum*, of south European origin, brought here by the Romans, cultivated on plots outside Sussex villages and towns, and found locally in the wild as an escapee.

All three contain a variety of powerful vermicidal principles; notably santonin, which the ancient Chinese purified from the Far Eastern wormwood *A. argyi*, and which is still used as a vermicide in modern medicine. The presence of powerful vermicides in these plants is no accident. They evolved to protect their possessors against the ravages of root, stem, and leaf-feeding nematode 'worms', but are equally effective against the closely related 'worms' which inhabit the human gut.

Not unnaturally, intestinal worms and snakes were classed together, and both linked with, or held to be incarnations of, the Devil; which is why on the one hand worms were credited with the snake's traditional diabolical cunning, and on the other why plants such as mugwort and absinthe genuinely effective against worms were invariably credited with powers against witchcraft and evil, and recommended for driving away snakes or as (probably ineffective) cures for snakebite.

This age-old confusion between intestinal worms and snakes in the minds of the rural population (and, until the 18th century, the learned too) is reflected in this passage from Richard Jefferies' *Wildlife in a Southern County*, 1879, describing gangs of cutters and stackers, harvesting by hand vast acres of hay:

'When the mowers have laid the tall grass in swathes snakes are often found in them or under them by the haymakers, whose prongs or forks throw the grass about to expose a large surface to the sun. The haymakers kill them without mercy, and numbers thus meet with their fate. The mowers who sleep a good deal under the hedges have a tradition that a snake will sometimes crawl down a man's throat if he sleeps on the ground with his mouth open. These snakes are bred in the stomachs of human beings from drinking out of ponds and streams frequented by water snakes...which snakes have been vomited by the unfortunate person afflicted with this strange calamity.'

Another popular Sussex treatment for worms involved swallowing 'worm-seeds', the seeds of the treacle mustard (see **Dacres of Herstmonceux)**.


# WOUNDWORTS

Many plants of the Sussex countryside are, or were, known as woundworts because of their remarkable blood-staunching wound-healing powers.

Two of the most highly valued in Sussex folk medicine were the marsh woundwort *Stachys palustris* and the hedge woundwort *S. sylvatica*. Both are recommended as wound-healing plants in the Anglo-Saxon *Leech Books of Bald and Cild*. Both, bruised and made into bandages, are recommended as dressings for cuts and bruises in the works of 16th-18th century local authors such as the agriculturist Leonard Mascal of Plumpton Place in the Tudor period, John Goodyer the Hampshire and West Sussex botanist, writing c1620, Edward Austin of Burwash, c1700, and William Borrer, the great Sussex botanist, c1810.

The herbalist Gerard first came across the healing virtues of marsh woundwort during a visit to Sussex:

'A very poore man,' he writes, 'in mowing did cut his leg with the Sieth, wherein he made a wound to the bones, and withal very large and wide, and also with great effusion of blood. The poore man crept unto this herbe which he bruised in his handes, and tied a great quantitie of it unto the wound with a piece of his shirt'.

Gerard was shown the wound and 'offered to heale the same for charitie which he refused, saying that I could not heale it as well as himself with his herbe; a very clownish answer I confesse, without thankes for my good will, whereupon I have named the herbe Clown's Woundwort.'

But the wound healed perfectly, and the man recovered without Gerard's help.

Once his hurt pride had healed too, Gerard applied marsh and/or hedge woundwort to every wound he was called on to heal. Even, and with success, to a shoemaker's assistant stabbed in the stomach and throat, 'a most mortall-seeming wound, in such sort that when I gave him drinke it came forth at the wound, which likewise did blowe out a candle'.

Other wild or herb garden plants used as woundworts in Sussex included pimpernel; salad burnet (*Poterium sanguisorba*, Latin *sanguis*, blood, *sorbere*, to absorb); its relative the Jacob's ladder, *P. caeruleum*, formerly known as Greek valerian, described by Turner as 'our common Valerian that the country folk use for cuts'; woad, once cultivated in East Sussex for its dye, and formerly common in the wild as an escapee; yellow flag; saw wort, 'woonderfully commended to be the most singular for wounds, ruptures, burstings, hernies, and such like'; twayblade; herb paris; Solomon's seal, also known locally in Sussex as Jacob's ladder; knapweed; elecampane; yarrow; golden rod; plantain, bugle; betony; and vervain.

Eva Brotherton, writing in 1927, says that there was 'nothing better for cuts and bruises than the petals of the Madonna lily, pickled in brandy, and laid on as a skin, which adheres to the injured part, healing and keeping it clean at the same time...'

The leaves of many of these woundworts contain defensive

tannins and phenols which evolved to coagulate the saliva of leaf-feeding insects (an insect whose saliva has coagulated is unable to feed and starves to death). They are equally good at coagulating blood to close blood-gushing wounds.

Some of the chemicals in the leaves of woundworts also sterilize the wounds they have closed. Marsh woundwort juice, for example, contains a powerful antiseptic oil. This oil, composed of bacteriocides and fungicides, evolved to protect the plant against bacteria, rusts and moulds. But it kills microbes of every description, including the ones that cause sepsis.

Though our sources are too patchy to allow any certainty, I have the impression that spiders' webs were the most widely used Sussex folk cure for wounds, because the cure was effective and easy to remember, and cobwebs were easy to obtain at short notice anywhere all year round. The use of woundworts was quite widespread – most 'wise women' seem to have known at least one wound cure based on the aplication of woundworts – but not as commonplace as the application of cobwebs. No doubt the reasons were that the appropriate plants might be more difficult to obtain at short notice (local in distribution or limited in growing season), and also their identification and use demanded a level of botanical knowledge possessed by some but not necessarily all members of the rural community.

# INDEX